Infectious Diseases of Poultry

Infectious Diseases of Poultry

Dr. S.V. Pandit
B.V.Sc. (Hons.) M.V.Sc. (Bacteriology)
(Bombay University)
P.G. (Denmark)

Dr. V.V. Deshmukh
B.V.Sc.& A.H.,. M.V.Sc.,Ph.D.
Veterinary Public Health & Epidemiology,
College of Veterinary & Animal Sciences,
MAFSU, Parbhani- 431 402 (Maharashtra)

International Books & Periodical Supply Service
(Publisher of Scientific Books)
38, NISHANT KUNJ, PITAM PURA MAIN ROAD
DELHI-110034 (India)
Phone : 011-27352078, Mobile : 09810146811, E-mail : hkjain1975@yahoo.com

Published by :

International Books & Periodical Supply Service

(Publisher of Scientific Books)
38, NISHANT KUNJ, PITAM PURA MAIN ROAD
DELHI-110034 (India)
Phone : 011-27352078, Mobile : 09810146811, E-mail : hkjain1975@yahoo.com

ISBN 978-81-93906-55-2

Composed, Designed & Printed in India

About the Authors

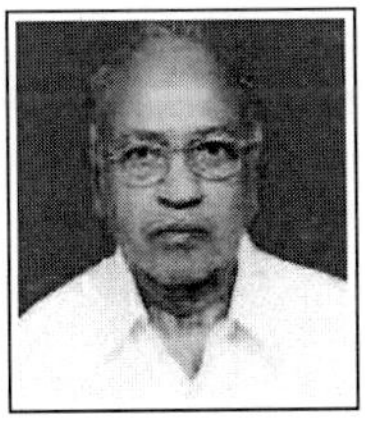

Dr. Sharadkumar Vishnu Pandit was born on 6th October, 1936. He obtained B.V.Sc. (Hons.) Degree from Bombay University and M.V.Sc. (Bacteriology, Pathology and Parasitology) of Bombay University of 1st Batch in the year 1962. He received 2 Years Training in Virology, Serology & Tissue Culture Techniques at various research centres, Pune (ICMR-Rockfellor Foundation's joint collaboration) between 1964-1966. He also participated in a Summer Institute in Immunology at I.V.R.I., Mukteshwar (U.P.) during 1971.

He had visited Denmark, Germany, U.K. Italy, France and Iran as DANIA Fellow for Advanced Post Graduate Training Programme in Foot & Mouth Disease Vaccine Production. He was also trained in Advanced Technology related to production and testing of Poultry Vaccines including Marek's Disease Vaccines during 1990 at Tri Bio Laboratories & Main Biologicals in U.S.A.

He worked in various capacities at Disease Investigation Section, Maharashtra State, Pune for a period of 14 years (1960-1974), which also includes his technical services as Assistant Professor at Agriculture University of Kolhapur & at Poultry Training Centre, Kolhapur, ICAR's Mucosal Disease and Blue Tongue Disease Research Schemes, Mastitis Research Schemes and All India Co-ordinated project on F.M.D. typing (ICAR).

He has a deep insight in production, testing and development of various viral and bacterial vaccines against important disease of Cattle, Sheep and Goats like H.S., B.Q. Foot and Mouth Disease, Rinderpest, Brucellosis, Multi-factorial clostridial infections, etc. while working as Manager, Research & Development at Bharatiya Agro Industries Foundation's Vaccines Production Centre at Wagholi, Pune for a period of long 14 years (1974-1988).

He worked extensively for a very long period of 18 years (1988-2006) in Development, Production, Testing and Field Application of Poultry Vaccines including those against ND, IB, IBD, Marek's Disease (Freeze Dried & Cell Associated Vaccines), Fowl Cholera, Fowl Spirochetosis, Fowl Coryza, Salmonellosis and lastly most important newly emerged Inclusion, Body Hepatitis/Hydropericardium Syndrome (IBH/HPS) at Ventri Biologicals, Division of Venkateshwara Hatcheries Group, Pune.

He was nominated as a member of committee for suggesting measures for control of emerging diseases of poultry under the Taskforce established by Govt. of India (ICAR, New Delhi) during 1998. They suggested (recommended) various measures for controlling newly emerging diseases like Avian Influenza, Gumboro disease, CAA and Reo virus infections of poultry in India. Establishment of projects of reference laboratories for Surveillance of these Disease Agents at some Regional places was the outcome of this committee including recommendations for strengthening HSDL, Bhopal (1998).

He worked as a member of scientific programme committee for 20th World Poultry Congress held at New Delhi, India during 2nd-5th September, 1996. He also acted as Chief Organiser of the technical sessions of this Poultry Congress on the subject "Poultry Health–Epidemidoge, Immunisation and Control Measures "at" Shahjahan Hall at Hotel Taj Palace.

He was a Technical Director of 2 Science films produced by Ventri Biological Division of Venkateshwara Hatchery, Pune, namely by i) Bio security programme for control of poultry diseases and ii) Production of poulry vaccines and their diluents, their reconstitution and vaccination techniques used in the field and vaccination schedules for Control of Poultry Diseases (1996). Similar film on production of live-stock diseases and their field use for control of livestock diseases was produced (Technical Direction) by the author (Dr. S.V. Pandit) and Dr. Devare when both of them were working at BAIF, Wagholi (1982).

He established fairly well-equipped laboratory facility at "Biospace" laboratories at Devachi Uruli, Pune with young enthusiastic Veterinarian Entrepreneur Dr. S.B. Salutgi (M.V.Sc.in Medicine) of Avians Trades, Pvt. Ltd. By 2012 for research work isolation and production of Bacteriophages for therapeutic use in control treatment of bacterial diseases of poultry and livestock like Salmonelosis and *E. coli* infections as well as strepto/staphylococcal infections of poultry and livestock. He also worked on use of *B. thuringenesis* for control of Domestic fly problem in poultry houses. He and S.B. Salutgi also developed technology for production of Silver Nano particles for control of Bacteriological problems in poultry (Salmonall/E.coli/Pasturella).The said work was done from November, 2009 to March, 2017.

He published few papers in technical journals including paper on "Development of Brucellalysate" for allergic test in Pigs (Dr. G.P. Sen of IVRI, Mukteshwar as Co-author). He participated in very large number of technical seminars of National / International importance and presented papers on subjects like Foot & Mouth Disease Virus typing, IBH/HPS Vaccine Development, Diagnostic Tests for Rinderpest and Mucosal Disease, Nephrotropic IB Vaccine, Diagnosis of Infections

Laryngio-trachaeitis. Author presented valuable papers on IBD Vaccine Development, IBH/HPS Vaccine Development in Symposia at IVRI as well as at World Poultry Science Congress held at New Delhi, in 1988. He also worked on newly emerging diseases like IBD, Chicken Anemia Agent (CAA) & Reo Virus Infections in Poultry.

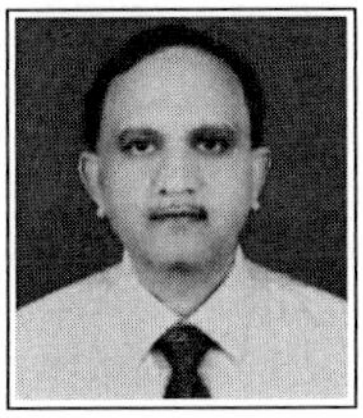

Dr. V.V. Deshmukh is working as Professor of Veterinary Public Health & Epidemiology in Maharashtra Animal & Fishery Sciences University at College of Veterinary & Animal Sciences, Parbhani. He started his career as Assistant Professor of Veterinary Microbiology at College of Veterinary & Animal Sciences, Udgir in the year 1987. He then worked as Junior Scientist at Animal Dissease Research Centre, Parbhani from 1994 to 2000. He was Associate Professor of Veterinary Microbiology from 2000 to 2008. He became Professor of Veterinary Public Health & Epidemiology in the year 2008.

He is having vast experience in disease diagnosis, surveillance, epidemiology, vaccinology of livestock and poultry diseases. He worked on FMD virus at ICAR, AICRP on FMD at DIS, Pune. Then, worked as Co-PI of ICAR Ad-hoc research project on 'Bluetongue in Ruminants' during 1994-1997. He was a PI of Parbhani Centre of ICAR, All India Network Programme on 'Bluetongue Disease' from 2001 to 2015. His major contribution was isolation of BTV-1. BTV-4 and BTV-18 from field outbreaks and a stakeholder in BT vaccine development under the programme.

He established Department of Veterinary Public health & Epidemiology at COVAS, Parbhani in the year 2008. A well-equipped Public health Lab was started with post graduate programme at the institute.

He has guided around 28 M.V.Sc. students, published large no. of research articles in national & international journals. He is a Ph.D. and M.V.Sc. paper setter, Thesis evaluator of no. of State universities and IVRI. He travelled to U.S.A., U.K. and Malaysia for professional assignments.His work has been recognized by Dr. D. S. Gorhe State Level Best Veterinary Teacher and Researcher Award of Senior Veterinarian Foundation, Pune (2014). Shyama Singh and Balamati Devi Memorial Award for Excellence in Animal Health Care and Cover by Indian Association for the Advancement of Veterinary Research (2016).

Preface

Poultry sector in India is broadly divided into two sub-sectors - one with a highly organized commercial sector with about 80 per cent of the total market share and the other being unorganized with about 20 per cent of the total market share. The egg production in the country has increased from around 83 billion nos. in 2015-16 to around 88 billion in 2016-17 registering a growth of about 6%. The per capita availability of egg has increased from 61 in 2013-14 to 66 in 2015-16. In 2016-17, it is 69. The broiler production is around 4.5 million tons which is approximately seven per cent more from last year possibly because of rising domestic demand for poultry meat. The growth in the broiler segment is expected to remain strong due to consumer preference for poultry, increasing income levels, and changing food habits. The live market sales of broiler meat still constitute more than 90-95 per cent of total volume of sales; the processed chicken meat segment comprises only about 5% of total production.

In recent times, Govt. of India has launched a massive Action Plan for Doubling Farmers Income by the year 2022. The Plan requires major emphasis on Health Sector. Infectious diseases of poultry play an important role in production. Prevention and control of infectious diseases require knowledge about various aspects of infectious diseases like aetiology, symptoms, postmortem signs, disease diagnosis, vaccination, etc. A lot of information about various infectious diseases of poultry is available now-a-days. However, information from experienced, senior professionals with their experiences may help in understanding poultry infectious diseases.

This book contains chapters on all major poultry diseases which are prevalent in India. The uniqueness of this book is that in addition to the description, valuable practical tips evolved out of experience of authors have been given. This makes the book valuable from field point of view. This book is meant for field veterinarians, students and professionals for reference. An attempt has been made to keep reader updated on historical facts, recent advances and practical hints on various infectious diseases of poultry endemic in the country. Poultry professionals are facing lots of problems due to emerging and re-emerging infectious diseases. This book will give an insight to the reader for better understanding of the problem.

Acknowledgement

The authors are highly obliged and thankful to Dr. M.R. Deo, of IVBP, Pune and Prof. (Dr.) R.D. Sadekar, M.V.Sc. Ph.D. Ex. Head of the Deptt. of Pharmacology of Krishi Vidyapeeth, Akola for their behind the curtain continuous help to write and publish this book and also the invaluable technical help in bringing this book project in actual reality.

Dr. S.V. Pandit, one of the author also takes this opportunity to express his gratitude towards his mentors, namely Late Dr. S.N. Sapre, its Director, D.I.S. (M.S.), Pune,Late Dr. S.G. Dixit, Ex. Dy. Director, IVBP, Pune, Late Dr. D.S. Gorha, Ex. Chief Executive, B.A.I.F.S F.M.D. Vaccine Project Wagholi, Dr. N.S. Dutt, Ex. General Manager, BAIFS, F.M.D. Vaccine Project, Wagholi,Late Dr. B.D. Survashe, Chief Executive, Ventri Biological of Venkateshwar Hatchery Ltd., Pune.

Dr. S.B. Salutgi, Director "Bio-space" Labotatory (Avians Drades Pvt. Ltd.), Pune, Dr. K.M. Pawar Madam, Ex. Director, NIV, Pune, Dr. S.V. Pandit has no suitable words to Express how he should acknowledge Late Dr. Manibhai Desai, Founder of BAIF, Wrali Kanchan,Late Dr. B.V. Rao, Founder of Venkateshwara Hatcherias Group, Pune without whose support his technical ambitions would not have materialized.

The authors are thankful to Mr. Milind S. Pandit and Mr. Manwatkar for their assistance in typing of this book.

Contents

Chapter 1

Ranikhet Disease

Ranikhet Disease (New Castle Disease)

Ranikhet Disease (RD) and New Castle Disease (ND), both are synonyms for one single deadly virus disease of poultry. The names are after the places, where the disease was first recorded.

Dr. T.M. Doyle reported the first outbreak from 'New Castle' in U.K., in 1926 while it was recorded from a hill station named 'Ranikhet' in Nainital district of present day Uttaranchal State for the first time in India. The reports of its occurrence poured in from all parts of the world then after. The credit for the ascending transition of the backyard poultry of yester years to the present day's mega-industry of poultry farming for meat and egg production should obviously go to the then scientists who evolved efficacious vaccines against this disease and also equally to the then field veterinarians who walked into the interiors of the country to vaccinate the birds, free of charge. Villagers were much elated to see their 'Vaccinated' birds survived while non-vaccinated succumbed to the disease in the face of outbreak. This was the 'direct proof' for the utility and popularity of the vaccine.

This demand for more and more vaccine compelled the then Govt. of Bombay to commence a special state level laboratory for R.D. vaccine in the year 1960, starting with liquid vaccine, which was started at Bombay and now located in IVBP, Pune-7 since then. Now it produces freeze dried RD (Mukteshwar) strain vaccine and 'Lasota strain' liquid vaccine.

The monograph on ND, a special Diamond Jubilee Publication, Scanning all Literature since 1926 on this subject was published by E. Alexander D.J. in 1980 entitled 'New Castle Disease' through 'Kluwer Academic Publishers', London, U.K. which is invaluable for researchers and students alike.

The virus: The virus belongs to the Para-myxo virus group PMV-I. There are separate PMV-1 to PMV-9 serotypes affecting variety of birds. The para-myxo virus group is further subdivided into 3 genera. The NDV belongs to 3rd genus, which consists of Influenza, Mumps and New Castle Disease virus (IMN group). The other 2 genera are:

i) Morbili virus – Measles, Rinderpest and Canine Distemper.

ii) Pneumo virus – Turkey Rhino-tracheitis and SHS.

The genome of NDV is single standard RNA with molecular weight of 5.2 to 5.7 x 10^6 daltons. It has the following set of NDV proteins (as per Page Analysis) (Fig. 1):

S. No.	Protein	Sr. No.	Protein	Remarks
1	NP	5	F1	Each protein Fraction eliciting its association with Specific function
2	NAP	6	F2	
3	M	7	HN	
4	Fo	8	L	

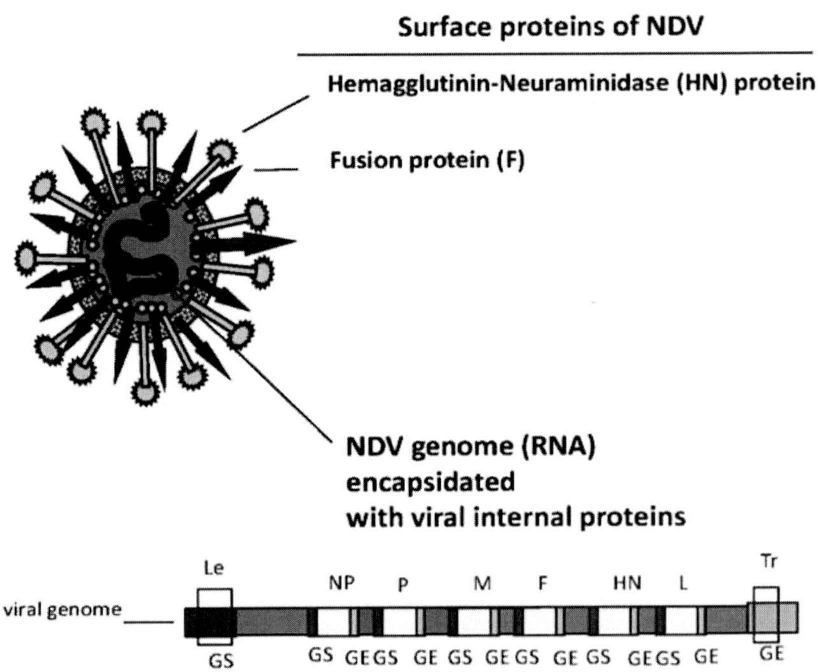

Figure 1: New castle disease virus

Hanson and Brandly (1955) proposed the classification of NDV isolates upon allantoic inoculation using mean dead time (MDT) as "velogenic", "mesogenic", and "lentogenic", based on chicken embryo mortality at <60 hours, 60-90 hours, or >90 hours, respectively. Other tests designed to differentiate strains directly assess clinical signs or death in infected birds, calculating a pathogenicity index. The most widely used test is the intracerebral pathogenicity index (ICPI) (Hanson, 1980). NDV infection is currently defined as a notifiable disease, if the virus has an ICPI of 0.7 in day-old chicks (*Gallus gallus domesticus*) (OIE, 2000b). An APMV-1 virus that does not meet the OIE definition for causing ND is referred to as a low-virulence APMV-1 or NDV.

Alexander (1988) has categorized ND patho-types as follows:

i) Viscero tropic Velogenic - Doyles

ii) Neuro tropic Velogenic – Beach's

iii) Mesogenic Velogenic – Beaudette's

iv) Lentogenic Velogenic – Hitchner's B, Lasota

v) Avirulent – Ulster type C.

This differentiation is based on Mean Death Time (MTD) of embryos. Pathogenecity involves inter play of multitude of factors, virus on one hand and the susceptible cell/host on the other.

The virus should have the communicability i.e. escaping from the infected cell, evading the host defenses; it should gain entry into new host cells and indicate infection. 'Pathogenecity' means virus replication and spread functions of vital organs. Viruses with 'tropism' for certain cells possess cleavability for activation of viral glycoprotein.

On the host side: (a) age of the bird, (b) susceptibility and/or immune status of the bird (c) route of infection, (d) magnitude of virulence and dose of infecting virus, (e) other environmental factors, such as humidity, temperature, wind flow/speed, rainfall and stress on the birds, are few of the factors influencing the outbreak.

Transmission

a) It was interesting to note the three prominent Panzootic Waves recorded by Alexander (1988) as follows:

First wave	1926 to 1942 south-east Asia/England
Second wave	1960 onwards including 1973 from Iraq to most of the countries through trade of psittacine birds.
Third wave	After 1980s through racing pigeon to poultry in almost all countries.

These outbreaks were the likely hood of infections from wild (feral birds) ducks, goose, pigeons and psittacine birds. Many of these birds, water fowls were found to be asymptomatic 'carriers'/reservoirs of the virus. Over 236 species of birds are known to be susceptible to ND virus and many more could be added to this list. Local unvaccinated birds also can either harbour the virus and/or on help, spread the virus.

b) Poultry houses in clusters and those poultry houses, accommodating adult chicken of various age groups under one roof, are more vulnerable to infection and its dissemination from the adults to chickens (adult birds vaccinated with mesogenic strain can cause infection in young chickens with little maternal antibody levels).

c) *Inter current* bacterial infections are the factors to aggravate the disease spectrum.

d) Human movements from one farm to another are also a source of each spread of infection. Hence, change of foot wear/apparels, etc. from one to the next farm has to be undertaken.

e) Transmission of infection is by ingestion and inhalation. Vertical transmission i.e. from parent via egg, to next progeny, is not recorded. However, if such eggs are extraneously contaminated with infected faeces, egg trays trucks, etc. Such embryos may show presence of virus. These embryos usually die much before hatching dates.

f) As stated earlier, infected water, feed, faeces, poultry products, vehicles carrying these poultry products all are potential source for carrying infection from one place/town/country to other place/town/country (e.g. II/III Panzootic waves mentioned previously). This underlines the stringency of legislation for transport (for trades) of birds/poultry products between countries. Quarantine measures, hence are absolutely necessary.

Diagnosis

a) **Clinical Diagnosis :** In velogenic per acute out breaks, eipzootology and the 'Sudden deaths' are the only indications. In less severe type, depression, prostration and greenish diarrhoea, edema (swelling) of the head and light mortality rate can be observed. Severe to moderate egg drop with shell less or soft shelled eggs are seen.

In moderately virulent pathotype, respiratory symptoms are observed with diarrhoea, torticollis of neck or paralysis of legs/wings in the 'nervous form' of the disease (Fig. 2).

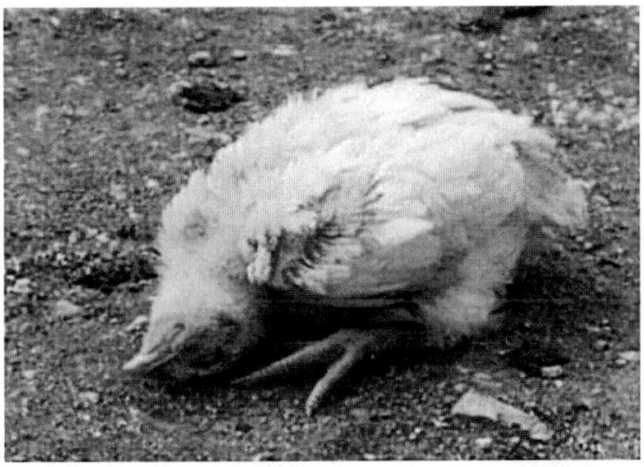

Figure 2: Nervous form of Ranikhet disease

Late in milder pathotype, there may not be any apparent clinical symptoms or at the most, in broilers, little respiratory distress is observed with loss of weight.

b) **Gross pathology:** Depicts pathognomic proventricular petechie on the 'tips' of proven tricular papillae and intestinal ulcers with bran like deposits on their borders.

c) **Laboratory Diagnosis:** There is as yet no accepted quick reliable *in vitro* test for ND. Virus isolation is still the only conventionally followed method. MDT (Mean Death Time) can further categorize the pathotype also. Intra cerebral pathogenecity test (ICPTest) in day old chicks or in 6 weeks old chicken are the other tests, in collaboration with 'MDT', to determine the ND strain, under investigation. H.I. tests are also complimentary. Monoclonal antibody tests (MAb) help to differentiate various strains of ND virus.

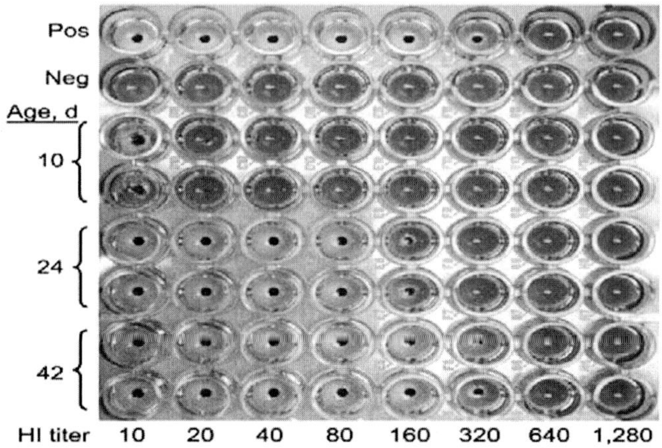

Figure 3: HI test for diagnosis of RD

Differential diagnosis : New castle disease virus being 'Pantropic' with various forms including, i) Classical Doyle's form with predominant 'enteric' affection, ii) Beach's neural form, iii) Hitchner's respiratory form, this disease can be confused clinically with various diseases and hence needs proper differential diagnosis.

Doyle's 'Enteric form' can be confused with 'Fowl plague' i.e. avian influenza. The proventricular lesions are pinpoint haemorrhages on the 'tips' of papillae of proventricular glands which are to be differentiated from haemorrhages surrounding the proventricular glands papillae all over the mucosa of proven triculus. Papillary haemorrhages of NDV can be confused with those of Gumboro disease but these can be differentiated by the formation of local band of such haemorrhages at the junction of gizzard and proventricular mucosa as against 'spread' of papillary tip haemorrhages all over the proven tricular mucosa in the case of ND.

The Neural form of ND is characterized by 'torticollis' of neck and lameness of limbs and wings while Avian Encephalomyelitis (AE) produces 'Lateral recumbence' and 'tremors' of limbs. The brain lesion of AE is characterized by 'Coughing' of lymphocytes in the space between lymphatic sinuses and enclosed blood vessel (known as space of Verco (lymphocytic accumulation) while the brain lesion of New Castle disease is characterized by 'proliferation' of the 'endothelial lining' of blood vessels in brain.

The respiratory form of New Castle disease shows haemorrhagic tracheitis, now-a-days, which can be confused with IB infection. Paired sera samples from acute phase of the disease followed by sera samples from the 'recovery' phase, if tested, simultaneously against NDV and IB by specific HAI tests or neutralization test will only be able to differentiate between ND and IB in such case.

Control : Control measures include strict: a) biosecurity, b) preventive vaccinations or c) legislation for import and export of poultry and their products and also of feral/psittacine/other birds.

All epizootological factors spreading infections are to be strictly controlled to stop ingress of infection. What measures one country has adopted may not be useful to other countries. Country has to envisage/legalize/ensure 'Rules and regulations' as per conditions of particular country.

Vaccines and Vaccinations

New Castle Disease (ND) outbreak, even though 1st officially recorded by Kraneveld in 1926 and Doyle in 1927, followed by recording of the same disease in India at Ranikhet village near Mukteshwar in Kumaon hill district, in U.P. in late thirties, it took year 1946 to develop Mukteshwar strain RD vaccine by Haddow and Idnani at IVRI, Mukteshwar. This vaccine development at IVRI was a big milestone in development of Poultry keeping in India. The early vaccines against ND were of 'partially attenuated (modified)' type with medium tire pathogenicity still existing in it (Also called as 'mesogenic' type).

Mesogenic Vaccine Strains

Amongst these 'mesogenic' types of vaccines, Mukteshwar strain (Haddow and Idnani, 1946) came after previous Hertfordshire (Herts) strain (Iyer and Dobson, 1940). Komorov or 'Hertford' strain (Komarov and Goldsmith, 1946) and Roakin strain (Budette *et al.*, 1949).

Roakin strain is naturally occurring mesogenic strain from United States while Komarov strain was developed by serial intracranial passaging of virulent virus through the ducklings in Hungary. Hertfordshire strain was obtained by serial passages in eggs and was in use in number of European countries while 'Mukteshwar strain' was generated by passaging of the field isolate in egg embryos and is the hottest amongst the mesogenic strains in the world. Original egg adopted 'Komorov' strain (mesogenic) was further passaged in CEF cell cultures by Ranipet Vaccine Institute of Tamil Nadu Government for reduction in its post-vaccinal neural reaction.

Lentogenic Vaccine Strains

It is a well known fact that all 'mesogenic' vaccine strains are highly immunogenic to the grower poultry birds of 6 weeks of age but they produce severe 'neural reactions' or the disease itself, if chickens younger than 6 weeks of age are 'exposed' or 'Vaccinated' with these mesogenic vaccine strains.

There were attempts to develop vaccine strains sufficiently milder enough for the use in younger chicks from day one to six weeks of age as the ND virus can produce the 'disease' in any age group of poultry after hatching. These milder strains of low pathogenicity are called as 'Lentogenic Strains'. They are also sometimes referred to as vaccine strains of B1 type (Allan, W.H and. Lancaster, J.E., 1978) ND (B_1) strain from USA (Hitchner and Johnson, 1948) and 'F' stain from U.K. (Asplin, 1952) and Lasota (Winter field *et al.*, 1952) are the 3 well known Lentogenic vaccine strains which are time proven for effective immunization of chicks from day one to six weeks of age.

Hitcher ND (B_1) also known as B_1 type B_1 strain in USA in naturally occurring mildest strain used for 'Priming' of the chicks from day one to day 7. Individually, the international standard for ND vaccine (live) was established in 1967 at Central Veterinary Laboratory, New Haw, Weybridge, Surrey, U.K. (Allan *et al.*, 1978). This strain was brought to India for vaccine production for use as 'Priming' of chicks by Ventri Biological Pvt. Ltd., Pune in 1998.

The F strain (Aspilin, 1952) from U.K. was another Lentogenic strain suitable for 'day old' vaccination (for up to 3 week old) chicken which was brought to India by IVRI Izatnagar and IVPM, Ranipet in early nineteen sixties.

Lasota strain was evolved by Winterfield *et al.* (1957) in USA. Late Dr. S.G. Dixit, the then Dy. Director of Institute of Veterinary Biological (IVBP), Pune, then proved to be 'Visionary' in bringing this promising Lasota strain to India in early nineteen sixties of 20th Century which was proved to be of immense value in effective control of RD in important poultry belts of Western India.

This vaccine was being produced as 'liquid' vaccine by the Govt. Laboratory. Paper was published in IVJ accordingly. However, the freeze dried version of Lasota was brought for commercial use by Ventri Biologicals, Pune in 1980 and BAIF vaccine project, Wagholi near Pune, in 1981, proved to be number one choice of poultry farmers in India for the control of ND.

The Lasota strain, being more 'invasive' than F strain, it is the strain of choice for bringing about effective post vaccinal immunological response in chicks with moderate to high maternal antibodies against NDV. This occurs due to the fact that Lasota strain can break through in spite of maternal antibody presence and reach the target cells situated in the Harderian glands and in the lymphoid aggregates spread in nasopharyngeal region and in submucosa along the upper respiratory tract including bronchi and trachea after occulo-nasal route vaccination and produce cellular immunity and local antibodies of IgA type. The immunity of chicks upto 6 weeks of age is dependent on this cellular and local antibody immunity. Hence, even through humoral antibody titres are not increased after Lasota vaccination after 'priming' the birds got protected against ND.

Recently, some multinational laboratories also introduced 'Clone 30' strain based vaccine (derived by cloning of Lasota strain by terminal dilution technique). This vaccine may be most suitable vaccine for the 'Biosecured' countries in Europe/Americas but in endemic countries like India where there are chances of frequent evolution of newer 'Pathotypic' mutants of the field strain of NDV due to 'resistance pressure' developed by antibodies in bird population by constant field strain exposures and vaccinations, its efficiency would be less assured.

'NDW' strain (van Eck *et al.,* 1991) is also another attenuated low passaged lentogenic strain which is claimed to be causing no post vaccinal reaction due to the precipitation of *E. coli* infection. However, it has not gained any popularity in India upto the date.

Queensland V-4 strain (Mazija *et al,* 2010) is another Lentogeic strain which is derived as 'temperature mutant' by exposure of Lasota strain to higher temperatures. This strain is claimed to be stable at room temperature. Thus, it can be used by incorporating the same in feed pallets stored at ambient room temperatures.

It is also claimed by certain multinationals that egg embryo based naturally trivalent 'entero-tropic' strain (e.g. :VG/GI strain) when given by oculo-nasal route, produces least mycoplasma precipitation and post vaccinal reactions.

However, it can be seen from the fact that ND (B1) strain is the most popular strain the world over for 'Priming' of chicks at day 1 to day 7 and Lasota is the strain of choice for boosting of immunity against NDV the world over. These claims of superiority of the above mentioned 'new strains' is only the 'marketing gimmick'.

Post Vaccinal Reactions

The route of live vaccination is important for the management of Post Vaccination Reactions in the chicks. It is known that Lasota strain is more 'invasive' than 'ND (B_1)' and 'F' strains. Hence, It (Lasota) can produce significant post vaccinal reaction, if the vaccine is applied by 'Spray' method, during the 'Priming' of chicks from day 1 to day 7. This happens due to stress on air sacs by fine droplets during spraying. If spray has 'coarse' droplets, this effect is low (This effect is known as 'bullet' effect). However, in India, spray vaccination is seldomly followed. Hence, if Lasota is applied by intra-occular or intranasal or drinking water route, this post vaccinal reaction is minimal or absent.

The Mukteshwar strain vaccine product's 'Neural Reactions' characterized by lameness in limbs and dropping of wings in 0.5 to 2 per cent of the birds, when the vaccine is given by intra-muscular or subcutaneous route in birds above 6 weeks of age. This is a 'normal' character of the mesogenic strain. However, this reaction becomes more intense and affects 5 to 8 per cent birds, if the birds are 'underweight' and if they are exposed to 'worm burden' in intestine or if they are harbouring significant 'coccidial infection'. The vitamin B deficiency is also responsible for this 'Neural reaction'. If the birds are having inadequate NDV antibody levels, then also there is severe 'Neural reaction'. If the birds are having inadequate NDV antibody levels, then also there is severe 'Neural reaction'. This problem can be tackled by :

i) Giving one more 'Lasota' booster vaccination at least 15 days prior to R_2B vaccination to build up sufficient NDV antibody levels.

ii) De-worming of birds ten days before R_2B vaccination.

iii) Use of anti-coccidials (Coccidiostats) in feed a week before vaccination.

iv) Use of anti-stress vitamin preparations like 'Stressvel'.

v) Administration of Vitamin B complex in drinking water a week prior to and after R_2B vaccination.

Pathogenic spectrum of the various vaccine strains for ND

The following information will give an idea about the 'Pathogenic spectrum' of the important vaccine strains against NDV. (Lancaster and Alexander, 1975):

Sr. No.	Strain	ICPI *	IVPI *	MDT (hours)
	A) Lentogenic strain			
1	Ulster Zc	0.0	0.0	>150
2	Queensland V_4	0.0	0.0	>150
3	Hitchner B_1	0.2	0.0	120
4	F	0.25	0.0	119
5	Lasota	0.4	0.0	103
	B) Mesogenic strains			
6	Komorov	1.40	0.0	69
7	Mukteshwar (R_2B)	1.44	0.68	46
8	Roakin	1.45	0.0	68
9	Herts 33	1.88	2.64	49

* ICPI – Intra Cerebral Pathogenecity Index in one day old chickens.
* IVPI – Intra venous Pathogenecity Index in 6 week old chickens.
* MDT – Mean Death Time "hours" after embryo infection with one minimal lethal dose.

Inactivated Vaccines : Hofstad, M.S. (1953) produced formalin inactivated egg embryo based 'tissue' vaccine followed by Grun and Hudson (1966). Later, Piercy *et al.* (1964) reported the use of aluminium hydroxide gel for adsorption of infected allantoic fluids. Extensive use of the oil emulsion based inactivated ND vaccines during epizootic in U.K., in 1970-71 is reported by Allan and Lancaster (1978).

The live vaccination programme in grower stage followed by inactivated, oil adjuvanted vaccines prior to laying can effectively bring about high antibody levels which can last long up to mid lay stage. Mid lay vaccination with inactivated oil adjuvanted vaccine will bring about long lasting immunity upto the end of economic egg laying period upto 72 weeks. Use of Lasota vaccination every 10 week's interval during this period can effectively bring about freedom from overt disease and drop in egg production.

Use of 'Lentogenic Virus' harvest with high titres is preferred to 'Velogenic' virus harvest for inactivated Vaccine production on the grounds of safety and efficacy.

The above mentioned 'Live vaccination programme' in grower stage followed by 'inactivated vaccination' programme in the breeder birds during laying phase throughout the economic lifespan mentioned above not only protect them during their lifespan but also bring about very effective transfer of NDV maternal antibodies in adequate quantum (high titre) in their progeny chicks (day old) which affords adequate protection to these chicks upto 6 weeks of age against NDV.

The above mentioned concept of use of inactivated vaccine in breeder birds for induction of maternal antibody (MAB) in commercial one day old chicks come to practice in India only in early nineteen eighties of 20th Century.

The following is the live and killed vaccination schedule generally followed especially for breeder birds:

Sr. No.	Name of Vaccine	Route of Vaccination	Day / Week of Vaccination
1.	ND (B1), live priming + ND (K)	Intraocular for live and subcutaneous 0.2 ml for killed vaccine	5th / 6th day
2.	Lasota live (Booster)	Intra ocular or drinking water	21st / 25th Day
3.	Lasota live (Repeat)	Drinking water route	35th day
4.	R_2B (Mukteshwar strain)	Intramuscular or subcutaneous route	6th / 8th week
5.	ND (Inactivated)	Intramuscular or subcutaneous route	12th / 13th week
6.	ND (Inactivated)	Intramuscular or subcutaneous route	16th /18th week
7.	ND (Inactivated)	Intramuscular or subcutaneous route	35th /40th week
8.	Lasota (Repeat) every 10th week after 18th week by drinking water route.		

Suggested Reading

Asplin, F.D. (1952). Immunization against New Castle disease with a virus of low virulence (Strain F) and observations on sub-clinical infections in partially resistant fowls. Vet. Rec. 64: 245.

Alexander D.J. (1980).New Castle Disease. Book published by Kluwer Academic Publishers, London, U.K.

Alexander D.J. (1988) Newcastle Disease : Methods of Spread. In: Alexander D.J. (eds) Newcastle Disease. Developments in Veterinary Virology, vol 8. Springer, Boston, MA.

Allan, W.H. and. Lancaster, J.E. (1978). Newcastle Disease Vaccines Their Production and Use. Rome, Food and Agriculture Organization of the United Nations.

Beaudette, F.R., Bivns, J.A. and Miller, B.R. (1949). Development of the mesogenic live vaccine Roakin. Cornell Vet. 39: 302-334.

Grun, J. and Hudson, C.B. (1966). Comparison of Beta-propiolactone whole embyo Newcastle disease vaccine (one strain) with abeta-propiolactone amino-allantoic New castle disease vaccine (four strain). Poult. Sci. 45(1): 159-164.

Haddow, J.R. and Idnani, J.A. (1946).Vaccination against New castle (Ranikhet) disease. Indian J. Vet. Sci.16: 45-53.

Hanson, R.P. and Brandly, C.A. (1955). Identification of vaccine strains of Newcastle disease virus. Science (122): 156-157.

Hanson, R.P. (1980). Newcastle disease. In: Hitchner S.B., Domermuth C.H., Purchase H.G., Williams J.E., editors. Isolation and Identification of Avian Pathogens. Kennett Square, PA: Arnold Printing Corporation. p. 63-66.

Hitchner and Johnson (1948). A virus of low virulence for immunizing fowls against Newcastle disease; avian pneumoencephalitis. Vet. Med. 43(12): 525-30.

Hrvoje Mazija, Stanko Èajavec, Neda Ergotiæ, Irena Ciglar-Grozdaniæ, Željko Gottstein, and William L. Ragland (2010). Immunogenicity and Safety of Queensland V4 and Ulster 2C Strains of Newcastle Disease Virus Given to Maternally Immune, Newly.

Hatched Chickens by Nebulization. Avian Diseases. 54(1): 99-103.

Hofstad M.S. (1953). Immunization of chickens against Newcastle disease by formalin inactivated vaccine. Am. J. Vet. Res. 14(53): 586-590.

Iyer, S.G. and Dobson, N. (1940). A successful method of immunization against Newcastle Disease of fowls. Vet. rec. 52: 891-94.

Komarov, A. and Goldsmith, L. (1946). Preliminary observation on the modification of a strain of Newcastle disease virus by intracerebral passage through ducklings. Veterinary Journal. 102: 212-218.

Lancaster, J.E. and Alexander, D.J. (1975). Newcastle Disease Virus and Spread. Canada Department of Agriculture, Monograph No. 11, Ottawa.

Van Eck J.H., Van Wiltenburg, N. and Jaspers, D. (1991). An ulster 2C strain-derived New castle disease vaccine: efficacy and excretion in maternally immune chickens. Avian pathol. 20(3): 481-495.

Winterfield, R.W., Goldman, C.L. and Seadle E.H. (1952). New Castle disease immunization studies IV. vaccination of chickens with B1, F and Lasota strains of Newcastle disease virus through drinking water. Poultry Science. 36: 1076-1088.

□□□

Chapter 2

Avian Infections Bronchitis

Avian infections Bronchitis (IB) is an acute highly contagious disease of the respiratory and /or uro-genital tract of chickens caused by a Corona virus, first identified in 1936, in the U.S.A., in Massatchusetts and reported in 1948, in Europe, where the disease spread rapidly since 1950s. IB continues to be a major cause of economic loss to the poultry industry worldwide, as it predisposes to secondary bacterial infections in the upper respiratory tract including naso-pharynx, facial sinuses and lacrimal tract. The economic losses are also due to severe 'egg drops' produced by IB infections which are generally of permanent nature. Of late, emergence of new genetic variants of 'nephrotropic' nature in IB virus resulted into high financial losses to the poultry farmers due to high early chick mortality on account of 'gout' problem.

Clinical signs

Classical symptoms of infectious Bronchitis (IB) inclue respiratory distress followed by rales, coughing, sinusitis and lacrimation in the affected birds. The disease can occur in young chicks from one week of age. However, uncomplicated cases of IB with respiratory syndrome were never detected in India. Generally, IB of chicks is found to be complicated with *E. coli* and mycoplasmosis which is detected as complicated chronic Respiratory Disease (cCRD) in young growing chickens.

It can be noted that Infectious Bronchitis was never detected in India prior to 1960. K.C. Verma reported "Mathura strain" of IBV in India for the first time in early nineteen sixties. Kumar worked under All India Co-ordinated Project for Respiratory Disease of Poultry at I.V.R.I., Mukteshwar in early nineteen sixties. He has mentioned in his report that respiratory disease observed in young chickens is complicated with multiple etiology including IB, mycoplasma and *E. coli,* etc. and hence, it can be properly described as "Respiratory Disease Complex (RDC)".

During Early Nineteen Eighties, we experienced an outbreak of Respiratory Disease characterized by facial oedema in layer grower birds in Hyderabad Poultry belt. This was presumed to be due to complication of IB infection with coryza infection. It is worth noting that IB inactivated vaccine was not available in India, in early eighties and IB live vaccine was being used in adult birds also for this reason. As use of live IB vaccine after 14 weeks of age of layer grower birds is not advisable due to possibility of infection of respiratory and reproductive tract with live IB vaccine strain. It is possible that vaccine strain (M-41/H-52) might be responsible for that incidence in Hyderabad. As a matter of fact "Egg drop" problems with production drop upto 30 per cent production after showing transient respiratory symptoms for initial short period in laying birds and production of 5 to 3 per cent eggs with corrugated shell surface was observed in IB infection of breeder and commercial layer birds, during 'Mid eighties'.

During the period from 1990 onwards upto 2005, on several occasions, we came across typical irreversible egg production drops (egg production of 80 to 90 per cent which is in rising phase or which has reached peak, suddenly dropped to 30 per cent or below) in layer flocks on breeder farm or commercial layer farm, showing presence of high percentage of thin shelled/cracked eggs and few shell-less eggs (Fig. 1). This results into poor hatchability and great losses to the breeder farm management or commercial salable egg production (Fig. 2).

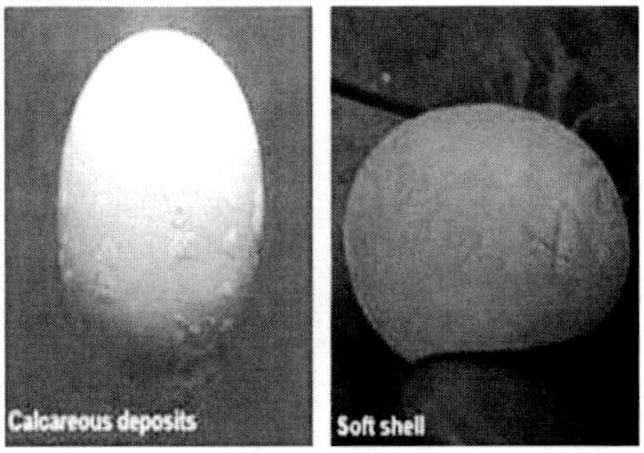

Figure 1: IBV infected egg defect

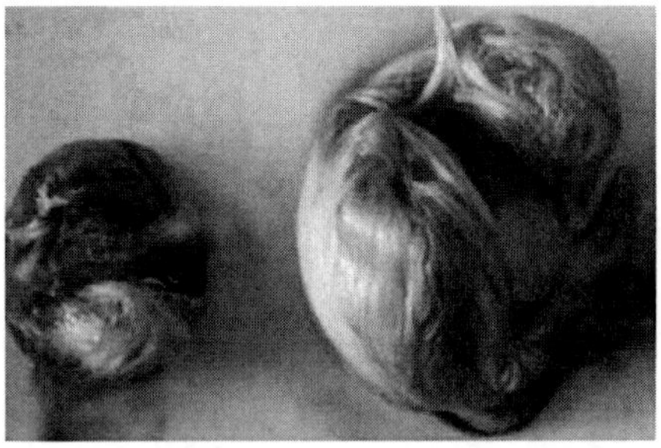

Figure 2: IBV infected embryo

Breaking of such thin shelled eggs and collection of their albumin-yolk contents in shallow dish reveals watery albumin in both the inner thick and outer thin layers of albumin (both layers become watery only). This phenomenon is diagnostic of IB infection in the bird.

As the "production drops" are irreversible in IB infection, continuation of the affected breeder or commercial layer flocks is futile and there is a need to discontinue and sale off the culled flock.

Gout (Nephritis) problem in broiler chicks due to IB infection

Deposition of urates in visceral organs including kidneys, spleen and liver (visceral gout) or in joints (Articular Gout) is due to multi-factorial reasons including nutritional, managemental, seasonal and infectious reasons in poultry as described in classical pathology books. However, during 2003 to 2005, large scale gout problems were experienced in Maharashtra, Andhra Pradesh (Hyderabad and Coastal Andhra) and Karnataka with high morbidity (50 to 70 per cent) and mortality (5.30 per cent) in younger age groups of commercial chicks from one day old to 3 week old. The causative agent was proved to be IB (Nephrotropic strain) virus. As a matter of fact, the author recorded incidence of gout (nephritis) in Talegaon (Maharashtra) in poultry layer birds in 1964, where in IB virus was isolated from kidney material by Dr. Kumar of All India Co-ordinated Project at IVRI, Mukteshwar which was reported as "Poona Strain" by him.

About the virus

IB is caused by Infectious Bronchitis Virus (IBV) which is a single stranded RNA virus belonging to the genus *Corona* virus in the family *Coronaviridae*. The envelop of the virus is associated with 3 proteins namely: i) large surface "Spike glycoprotein" (S) which is elevated into 2 sub units S1 and S2 ii) Small membrane glycoprotein (M) and iii) a very small non-glycosylated protein (SM or E) which is encoded by gene 3. The RNA genome is coated with the nucleo-capsid protein (N). It is considered that the changes in "S" protein gene (especially S1 part) are responsible for enabling field strains to break through vaccine induced immunity as S1 exhibits the most extensive sequence variation and forms the epitopes that induce virus neutralizing and haemagglutination inhibiting antibody (Cavanagh, 2005).

Virus neutralization tests in egg embryos or by using 'Ciliary stasis test' have been traditional technique for identification of strains of

IBV and assigning them groups or serotypes. Since 1956, new serotypes of IBV have been reported in various continents. To date, over 50 different serotypes have been detected in the world. Most important serotype strains can be named as: 1) Massachusetts strain 2) Arkansas strain, 3) Connecticut strain. All these being North American original strains: Baudette strain is a very highly embryo adapted Massachusetts type strain. The other most persistent serotypes and variants recorded in the world are:

a) AZ 23/74 Mostly Nephropathogenic strain reported from Italy (1974), prevailing for nearly 25 years and now missing.

b) D-274 and D-1466 with respiratory tropism reported from Netherlands (1983)

c) CR 88121 reported from France (1986) and 793B or 4/91 reported from U.K. (1991) which is mostly respiratory.

d) AZ-27/98 or Fa-6881/97 respiratory and or nephropathogenic (1997) reported in Italy.

e) PV strain which is Nephropathogenic isolated in 1965 from Italy.

f) 'T-z' strain which is highly Nephotropic reported from Australia.

g) H-56 and H-120 are Massachusetts type strains which are embryo adapted vaccine strains from Holland (Netherlands), the Number 56 and 120 indicate embryo passage level.

It should be noted that many field isolates of D-274 and D-1466 types from Netherlands and CR-88121 from France were found to be having a character of high embryo adaptation and they could be isolated in egg embryos during the first two passages only indicating that these must be vaccine strains only but have reverted back to virulence in the field quickly.

It is a well known fact that the IBV exhibits extensive antigenic variation which has led to the identification on many serotypes. Molecular studies have shown that the new virus serotype or 'Variant' can emerge as a result of only few changes in amino-acid composition in the S1 part of virus spike protein and of particular virus replication modem (discontinuous transcription), with the majority of the genome remaining unchanged. The sharing of so many antigens in different virus isolates might more or less be able to provide complete protection against challenge with viruses belonging to different serotypes. This explains how Massachusetts serotype M-48 vaccine strain/H-120 vaccine strain can provide protection against a broad spectrum of field virus serotype strains.

Diagnosis and serotyping: Serum virus Neutralization test using hyper immune (Polyclonal) serum produced against known IB is used for identification of field IBV isolates. Similarly, antigen capture ELISA test or Haemagghtination Inhibition (HAI) test using chicken erythrocytes treated with Neutralization dose of enzyme lipase procured from *Clostridium perfringens* and then adsorbed with IBV (known) and paired sera samples (acute stage and recovery stage) from the infected bird can be used for detection of IB antibodies. If the titer of recovered serum sample is higher than acute stage serum sample, the bird is diagnosed to have suffered from IB infection. All the 4 tests, namely serum virus neutralization test in embryonated eggs or 'ciliary stasis' test on tracheial/oviduct organ culture and HAI test as well as 'antigen capture' ELISA test can be used for diagnosis of IB but these tests are unable to detect the "serotype" specific IB antigens.

For serotyping only monoclonal "epitope" specific serum virus neutralization test will have to be used, using embryonated eggs. A number of reports have addressed the development and application of IBV monoclonal antibodies (MAbs). Mockett *et al.* (1984) reported production of 2 MABs to S1 protein of IBV strain Mass-41 which neutralized the virus at high dilutions. Koch *et al.* (1986) showed that MABs to N and M proteins could be quite broadly reactive while those specific to S2 displayed less cross reactivity. Karaca *et al.* (1992) produced serotype specific MAbs to 3 North American serotypes (Arkansas, Connecticut and Massachusetts). Nagi *et al.* (1991) used those Mabs to develop an antigen capture ELISA for typing of IB isolates.

Polymerase Chain Reaction (PCR) and Restriction Fragment Length Polymorphism (RFLP) analysis: Lin *et al.* (1991) used these 2 techniques for IBV isolate typing. (please see an article by S.A. Nagi entitled "Advances in Diagnostic Techniques for Avian Infections Bronchitis appeared in XX World Poultry Congress, 1996 (India) Vol. 2 Proceedings, pp.369-373) and an article entitled polymerase chain reaction and sequencing for avian disease diagnosis by D. Cavanagh *et al.* (1996) on pp. 487-495 under the same proceeding's volume.

However, as there are very large number of 'Serotypes' existing in nature and as IB virus is highly 'mutagenic' in nature, as already explained under the paragraphs included in the description 'about the virus' the 'Immuno types' or 'Protecto types' are important for consideration of vaccine production against a battery of serotypes existing in the particular country or area. Detection of protectotype needs usage of 'Cross protection tests' *in vivo* (in host species i.e. birds). Number of groups of birds are vaccinated with the vaccine produced from one specific vaccine strain (presumably protectotype) and different vaccinated groups are individually challenged with different serotype strains. The battery of 'Serotypes challenged' groups which withstand to the immunity produced by the presumed protectotype vaccine are supposed to belong to that 'protectotype'. Thus, mass-41 strain/H-120 protectotype can provided full protection against a number of serotypes. These serotypes are supposed to belong to only one protectotype.

Vaccines and Vaccinations

In India, as large number of field isolates have shown their tendency to get included in 'Massachusetts' protectotype, vaccine strains M-48 and H-120 are being used for protection against IBV infection since 1980-81 onwards.

Generally, IB vaccination is carried out using live IB vaccine at day old stage by intra ocular route followed by drinking water route vaccinations at 4th week, 8th week and $12^{th}/13^{th}$ week age (live vaccine). IB (Killed vaccine) at $17^{th}/18^{th}$ week is generally used at prelay stage in breeding blocks or sometimes in commercial layer flocks for affording protection upto midlay stage to the breeding flocks as well as for maternal antibody transfer to their commercial layer/broiler chick progeny which can get passive MAB protection upto 3 weeks of age against IB infection. This is followed by 'Midlay vaccination' in breeder birds at 35 to 40 weeks of age which covers protection to them and their progeny upto the disposal of flocks by 60 to 80 weeks.

During early sixties to early eighties period, no IB vaccine was being produced in India and people were forced to use IB live vaccines even after 14th week of age. This was a dangerous practice and which might be responsible for evolution of variant strains in the field by 'point mutations' in spike proteins. This might be a reason for occurrence of frequent 'egg drop' problems described in India from

1990 onwards upto 2005-06, especially in breeder flocks inspite of following of IBV (inactivated) vaccination programme undertaken during that period by breeders (prolong and midlay vaccinations).

The incidences of Nephrotropic IBV infections with gout in early age group chicks (one day to 3 weeks age), especially broiler chicks occurred in India twice on large scale, i.e. during 2000 to 2001 once and then again during 2003 to 2005. Both the time, new nephrotropic IBV strains which had very little 'relatedness' with each other was found to be present and hence, only after production of experimental inactivated IBV vaccines using the homologous field IBV Nephrotropic virus isolates for vaccination of breeder flocks could halt the incidences of gout in their commercial progeny.

Suggested Reading

Cavanagh D., Naqi S.A. (1997). Infectious bronchitis. In Calnek B. W., Barnes H. J. and Beared C. W.. Diseases of Poultry. 10th Edn., Ames: Iowa State University Press. Chap. 17: 11-526.

Cavanagh, D. (2005). Coronaviruses in poultry and other birds, Avian Pathol. 34: 439–443.

Karaca, K., Naqi, S. and Gelb Jr., J. (1992). Production and characterization of monoclonal antibodies to three infectious bronchitis virus serotypes. Avian Dis. (36): 903-915.

Koch, G., Hartog, L. and Kant, A. (1986). Antigenic differentiation of avian bronchitis virus variant strains employing monoclonal antibodies. Isr. J. Vet. Med. (42): 89-97.

Lin Z., Kato A., Kudou, Y., Kudou Y. and Ueda S. (1991). Archives of Virology 116: 19. https://doi.org/10.1007/BF01319228

Mockett, A.P.A., Cavanagh D., Brown, T.D.K. (1984). Monoclonal antibodies to the S1 spike and membrane proteins of avian infectious bronchitis coronavirus strain. Massachusetts M41.J. Gen. Virol. (65): 2281-2286.

Zanella A., Ceruti R. and Gavazzi L.(2005). Infectious Bronchitis: An Overview of European Epidemiological Situation Report of 54th Western Poultry Disease Conference, pp. 1-2.

❑❑❑

Chapter 3

Infectious Laryngo Tracheitis

Infectious laryngotracheitis (ILT) is a respiratory disease, principally of the upper respiratory tract. Following natural infection, disease signs appear in 6-12 days (Jordan, 1966). Peracute, subacute and chronic (or mild) forms of the disease may occur (Tripathy, 1998; OIE, 2000b). The peracute form is characterised by sudden onset and rapid spread with high morbidity. In such outbreaks, mortality may exceed 50% (Jordan, 1966). Affected birds show characteristic clinical signs associated with respiratory distress. Birds may sneeze, gasp or cough, sometimes producing clots of blood. Gurgles, rattles and rales may be heard due to tracheal obstruction.

In the subacute form, morbidity is again high, but mortalities are typically lower, varying from 10% to 30%. The spread of disease and the development of clinical signs occurs more slowly, with respiratory signs observed for some days before deaths occur. Affected birds may also show conjunctivitis with associated lacrimation and swelling of the infra-orbital sinuses. The chronic/mild form of ILT may be seen subsequent to peracute and subacute outbreaks or as a distinct disease entity. Mortality rates are typically 1-2%, with losses occurring over a period of months. Affected birds may be unthrifty, with bouts of gasping and coughing accompanied by nasal or oral discharges. A considerable drop in egg production may also be seen in laying birds (Jordan, 1966).

Infectious Laryngo tracheitis (ILT) is an acute or subacute infectious disease of chickens caused by herpes virus of poultry.

Clinical disease is characterized by gasping, coughing, rattling and extension of neck during inspiration. Anorexia occurs during the disease and there can be exudation of blood stained cough through mouth and beak.

Mortality can occur upto 50% in the affected flock, which can be due to occlusion of trachea by haemorrhagic exudation.

Incubation period of the disease may be from 5 to 12 days, and usually the disease subsides after about 2 weeks. Subacute disease can occur due to milder strains of low virulence and mortality will be negligible or absent. The egg drop can occur slightly.

About the Virus

Gallid herpesvirus 1, better known as infectious laryngotracheitis virus (ILTV), is a member of the genus *Iltovirus*, subfamily *Alphaherpesvirinae* of the family *Herpesviridae* (Davison *et al.*, 2009). ILTV is a pathogen of the respiratory tract of poultry, producing peracute, subacute and chronic or mild disease outbreaks (Guy and Garcia, 2008). All ages of poultry are susceptible to infection, and mortalities in peracute outbreaks may exceed 50%. Respiratory signs predominate, although decreased egg production may also occur in layers. Virus persists in a latent state in recovered birds, being shed intermittently. Where the virus is present, management often relies on the use of live attenuated vaccines. Vaccinal strains also establish latency and can be subsequently shed. Vaccinal strains have the potential to revert to virulence, and vaccinated and non-vaccinated birds should, therefore, not be mixed.Typical POC lesions can be seen on choreo-allantioc membrane of the susceptible chicken egg embryos, if the suspected tracheal exudate material is inoculated in 9 to 12 days old incubated egg embryos by choreo-allantoic route and histo-pathological examination of the same reveals intra-nuclear inclusions, which are characteristics of herpes virus (*Gallid herpes virus I*).

Epidemiology of the disease

ILTV is predominantly a pathogen of chickens (Bagust and Guy, 1997). Although all ages are susceptible, the most characteristic signs of disease are seen in adult birds. Disease has also been reported in peasants and peafowls (Cranshaw and Boycott, 1982). Experimentally induced infection of young turkeys has also been reported associated with an age-related resistance (Winterfield and So, 1968). Other species, including closely related galliforms are refractory to infection.The recovered birds remain carriers of the herpes I virus of ILT throughout life and can spread the disease to susceptible birds. The latent virus reactivates under stress. Mechanical spread of the disease can occur due to the practice of spread of litter in pastures.

It is well known that vaccinated birds and non-vaccinated birds should not be mixed, as vaccine virus can be reversed back to virulence in non-vaccinated birds.

Lesions of the Disease

The disease is characterized by prominent postmortem lesions, such as yellow caseous exudate or hollow caseous casts in trachea. Histo-pathological finding of presence of intra-nuclear inclusion bodies in tracheal epithelium during initial phase of the disease with necrotizing epithelial tissue in the tracheal cast, infiltration of mononuclear cells is also observed in inflamed tracheal tissue section. The diptheritic form of fowl pox can be diffrentiated from ILT by observing intracytoplasmic inclusions in tracheal epithelial cells as against intra-nuclear inclusions of ILT.

Control of ILT infection : The disease can be effectively controlled by vaccination and even vaccination in the face of the outbreak can be undertaken to help reduction of further morbidity and mortality. Strict biosecurity and disinfection program is helpful in reduction of the severity of the disease.

Most of the vaccine strains are modified live isolates and are administrated by eyedrop method. ILT vaccine strains used in live vaccine are produced on 9 to 12 day old egg embryos innoculated by choreo-allantoic membrane route (dropped membrane) or produced on cell cultures of SPF egg origin.

Indian Scenario: The disease (ILT) was not prevailing in India up to mid-nineteen sixties. One of the Authors (S.V. Pandit) recorded first incidence of ILT in India (or atleast in Maharashtra) in 1964 at a poultry farm near Boat Club, Pune (belonging to Catholic Church) in the chickens received from M/s Arbor Acres (Talegaon) Hatcheries. The source of the outbreak traced back to the ILT vaccination (which was not practiced in Pune elsewhere in those days) of chick's batch received from Arbor Acres hatcheries and mixing of these chicks with previous unvaccinated birds on the recipient's farm (reported in Indian Microbiological Society, Pune's Conference, 1965). However, there were no other official outbreaks of ILT detected in India after this sporadic incidence upto the recent past. The above mentioned outbreak was confirmed by histo-pathological report (Intranuclear inclusions) by Prof. B.L. Purohit of Bombay Veterinary College.

Recently, after official occurances of Avian Influenza in India, in late 2004 (Maharashtra), many outbreaks of haemorrhagic Tracheitis were attributed to ILT infection instead of to AI by Venkateshwara Group Scientists (personal communications).

During very recent incidances in 2017, Poultry Industry in Hyderabad, Telangana State suffered from heavy losses due to deaths occurring because of haemorrhagic tracheitis outbreaks attributed to ILT confirmed histo-pathologically (personal communication during field investigations).

Suggested Reading

Jordan, FT.W. (1966). A review of the literature on infectious laryngotracheitis (ILT). Avian Diseases, 10: 1-26.

OIE, (2000b). Avian infectious laryngotracheitis. In: Manual of Standards for Diagnostic Tests and Vaccines, edition 4. Paris, France: Office International des Epizooties, 711-717.

Tripathy, D. N. (1998). Infectious laryngotracheitis. In:Laboratory Manual for the Isolation and Identification of Avian Pathogens, edition 4. Pennsylvania, USA: American Association of Avian Pathologists, 111-115.

❑❑❑

Chapter 4

Emergence of Very Virulent Infectious Bursal Disease (VVIBD) in India: Its Prevention and Control

Infectious Bursal Disease (IBD) was first described in 1957 by Cosgrove (1962) in the country town of Gumboro, Delaware, in Delmarva region of U.S.A., as a condition causing high mortality with lesions consisting of Nephrosis, bursal oedema and necrosis in broilers. Hence, the commonly used term 'Gumboro Disease'.

The disease was later on recorded in Europe and many other countries throughout the world. Even though the classical form of IBD was recognized by various scientists including Mohanti *et al.* (1971) in India since 1971, this viral disease was confirmed by isolation and identification of the virus in Bombay-Pune Poultry belt by Dr. Ajinkya, S.M. and Dr. Survashe, B.D. in 1976-77.

The classical IBD was characterized by moderate mortality (5 to 10% in layer birds and 3 to 5% in Broilers), but more significant was immune-suppression caused by severe damage to follicles of Bursa of fabricious which is the 'nursery' of B cells responsible for humoral immunity production in the birds.

The incidence of classical IBD in Bombay-Pune belt in 1976-77 brought about increased incidence in coccidiosis and failure of immune response to ND Lasota vaccinations as a result of immune-suppression after subclinical exposures to classical IBD virus. This situation prevailed up to 1991-92.

Emergence of VVIBD

Emergence of very virulent form of IBD (VVIBD) characterized by high morbidity and mortality was first reported in Belgium and Netherlands in 1987, followed by its incidences in France, Germany and U.K. by 1981-1991 (Chettle *et al.*, 1989, Vandenburg *et al.*, 1991).

In August, 1990, outbreaks of acute IBD were recorded in Western Japan (Nunoya *et al.,* 1992). Middle East, Egypt, South Africa, Nigeria and Asia Pacific nations including Japan, Indonesia, Phillipines, China and Bangladesh were reported to be affected by 1991-92. Incidence of VVIBD was reported in Nepal by August, 1992 (VH group investigations) which was later on confirmed by IVRI workers (Sah *et al.,* 1995). It is interesting to note that VVIBD has not been reported from U.S.A., wherein incidence of classical IBD as well as highly Immuno-suppressive antigenic variants (Rosenberger's Variants) were recorded (Craft *et al.,* 1990, Ismail and Saif, 1991).

Emergence of VVIBD in India

Incidence of very virulent form of IBD (VVIBD) was reported from Hugali and 24 Paragana districts of West Bengal during November, 1992 for the 1st time in India. This incidence was involved in the initial investigations of this new problem in Hugali and further follow-up investigations in eastern coasts and south India during 1992-93.

It was reported by the farmers that the source of the 1st incidence of VVIBD in Calcutta Poultry belt originated from affected chicks received from Nepal. The disease incidence gained the proportion of an 'Epornitic' (epidemic) and the wave of VVIBD appears to have spread from West Bengal to Vishakhapattanam (January, 1993), Hyderabad (Jan, 1993) Chittor, Nellore (Jan, 1993) and Namakkal (March, 1993), followed by incidence in Bangalore and Mysore belts (March-April, 1993), and later on in Maharashtra (April–May, 1993). Subsequently the disease spread to the other parts of the country including Gujarat (August, 1993), Punjab-Haryana (September, 1993), M.P. (1993) and U.P. (1994-95).

In the initial Phase, the VVIBD virus could sweep through thickly populated poultry belts like Hyderabad, Namakkal and Vijaywada and took a very heavy toll in layer birds, as the population of the poultry birds in the country was poorly immunized against IBD prior to 1992 (8.6% breeder birds and 1.8% commercial layer birds were only immunized) and hence, the disease could take a very heavy toll in layer birds. Spike mortality ranged from 40 to 80% due to IBD alone and enhanced upto even 90% when mixed with ND or *E. coli* infections (Survashe and Pandit, 1994 and Anonym, 1995) or when mixed with IBH/HPS syndrome (Gupta, 1994). Mortality in broiler birds ranged from 20 to 30 per cent in the 1st phase of VVIBD.

In the beginning, outbreaks occurred in the age group of 7th to 12th weeks age in layer birds and 6th to 7th weeks in broiler birds. Subsequently, there was a shift to the left in IBD incidence age wise and outbreaks started occurring in earlier age groups (4 to 6 weeks) with layer birds, mortality ranging from 10 to 25% and broiler mortality from 2 to 10%. Shift to the left in age group can only be explained by the fact that about 60% to 65% farmers from the thickly poultry populated areas desparately used 'Induced Bursa' practice at about 18 days age (used IBD infected bursa triturate containing drinking water), resulting in low mortality by 'Induced IBD' at the age of about 4th week, but this led the flocks to become susceptible to secondary infections (bacterial/viral) due to severe immune suppression caused by induced IBD.

Indiscriminate use of IBD intermediate plus i.e. 'Hot IBD' vaccine in birds for more than 2-3 generations or in the birds at an early age (3 to 5 days age) with low maternal immunity was responsible for secondary bacterial/viral infections leading to heavy economic losses to the farmers.

Epidemiology

Large scale movement of vans with contaminated egg trays, culled birds from infected premises to the inter and intra state markets and back to non-infected farms were the major reasons for the spread of VVIBD throughout the country. Hence, the name 'High way disease'. Improper disposal of infected carcasses in thickly populated poultry belts was equally responsible for fast spread of the infections. The practice of utilizing used litter, basket brooders in broiler premises helped in perpetuation of 'Cyclical infection' in replacement broiler flocks. Inadequate biosecurity and disinfection measures on the farms (equipments, waterers, feeders and farm personnel) between two cycles of broiler replacement were responsible for unending cycling of infections on the farm premises. IBD virus can remain viable on the farm premises upto 60 days or more, as it is thermo-stable virus. Even veterinarians, poultry consultants and vaccinators were responsible for 'mechanical spread' of infection from farm to farm. Re-use of gunny bags from infected premises for supply of feed to new farms resulted in dissemination of infection. Rats, beetles, and insects were also incriminated as mechanical carriers of infection from flock to flock and farm to farm.

In absence of exact figures of mortality and morbidity, the economical losses could not be calculated but considering 40-80% mortality in layer flocks, losses must be enormous.

About the virus

The virus belongs to the *Birnaviridae* Family and has a double stranded RNA. It has 5 viral proteins (VP) of which VP_2 and VP_3 have neutralizing epitopes. It is relatively resistant to a variety of environmental conditions and it was reported to have survived for 122 days in a house after depopulation of an infected flock. It is also resistant to commonly used disinfectants. It is highly contagious and has been isolated from insects and beetles in poultry houses. The control of virus is based on vaccination with homologous virus type and bio-security measures, which are complimentary to vaccination.

Virus types

Cosgrove (1962) reported IBD for the first time in cases of avian nephrosis. Only one antigenic type (Serotype-1) was recognized until in 1980. The serotype-2, which was distinct from serotype-1 antigenically and immunologically, was reported by Mc Ferran *et al* (1980). The serotype-2 viruses were isolated in USA from chickens and turkeys by Lukert and Saif (2003).

Saif *et al.* (1987) reported a major antigenic variant of serotype-1 that was isolated from broiler chicks with high levels of maternal antibodies. The variant was associated with severe disease outbreaks in the Delmarva Peninsula in the early nineteen eighties. Later similar viruses (varieties of serotype-1) were isolated by Rosenberger and Snyder laboratories.

Studies on antigenic relatedness of several field and vaccine strains of IBDV isolated before 1984 (classic or standard) and some variant strains isolated after 1984 demonstrated the high antigenic diversity of the virus. In the antigenicity studies, polyclonal antibodies were used in a virus neutralization test. This proves to be a good '*in vitro*' system that provides a reasonable prediction of the immunogenicity of the virus. In immunogenicity tests, chickens were used and the results indicated reasonable agreement between *in vitro* antigenicity and *in vivo* immunogenicity studies. This agreement was not evident, when other serological tests like 'ELISA' were used.

Based on above studies, three major antigenic and immunogenic types are currently (year 2004) recognized. These are: 1) serotype-1, 2) variant serotype-1, 3) Serotype-2 viruses. Subtypes of these 3 major types are also recognized. Classical serotype-1 viruses will induce full protection against homologues viruses and partial protection against variant viruses. Variant viruses provided full protection against both the homologous and the classical viruses. Serotype-2 viruses provide no protection against serotype-1 viruses. In 1985, a major new pathotype of the virus recognized as very virulent (VVIBD) was described in Europe which spread all over the world except in USA. The VVIBD which is described in India since 1992 is pathotypically antigenically and immunologically similar to the European VVIBD and is similar to classical serotype-1 virus but pathotypically different from the same.

Antigenic structure of field and vaccine viruses

Monoclonal Antibody studies in Rosenberger's and Snyder laboratories in USA could reveal the antigenic differences on 'epitope' level between the classical serotype-1 virus and VVIBD field virus which is, even though pathotypically different from it (serotype-1) is serologically same as serotype-1. They showed presence of antigenic epitopes Nos. 8-m, 10, 179, R-63, B-69 and B-29 on the surfaces of both classical serotype-1 and VVIBD serotype-1 viruses. However, B-69 epitope is quantitatively higher in 'quantum' on VVIBD than on serotype-1 and epitope-21 is additionally present on the surface of VVIBD while it is totally absent on 'serotype-1' classical virus. High quantum of B-69 epitope on VVIBD makes it more immune suppressive and presence of epitope No.21 on VVIBD provide high pathogenecity to the same. (This pathotypic character is absent in classical serotype-1 virus as there is absence of epitope-21 on it).

It is worthwhile to note that IBD (Lukert strain) vaccine works well against classical serotype-1 field virus because it bears epitopes Nos. 8, 179, R-63, 10, B-69 in almost similar quantum as on classical sero type-1 field virus and epitope No. B-69 is present on IBD (Lukert vaccine strain) on its surface, as in case of classical serotype field virus, though in small quantum. However, it is interesting to note that epitope-21 is totally absent on the surface of IBD (Lukert) vaccine strain and B-69 epitope is even though present on it, the quantum of it is so insignificant that it cannot take care on very high quantum of B-69 epitope present on VVIBD. Hence, the Lukert vaccine strain can't afford enough protection of VVIBD.

It can be noted that IBD (Intermidiate) vaccine strain can provide slightly better protection against VVIBD field strain because it has higher quantum of B-69 epitope present on the surface as compared with IBD (Lukert) strain. However, IBD intermediate plus vaccine strain has still higher B-69 epitope presence, and it has small quantum of additional '21' No. epitope presence which makes it to match with field VVIBD strain more as compared with IBD Intermediate Vaccine Strain.

Clinical symptoms and post mortem findings in VVIBD infection

Affected birds look dull, show ruffled feathers and many remain in prostrate position, emiting creamy coloured diarrhoea and some may tremble. The daily mortality follows a specific pattern called as 'spike' mortality.

Postmortem of affected birds revealed severe ecchymotic type of 'muscular haemorrhages' on the breast and thigh muscles. Prominent enlargement of bursa of fabricious with gelatinous yellow transudate covering the serosal surface is seen and presence of mucous with or without blood inside the bursa in the acute stage of the disease also observed. Occasionally 'regressed' bursae are observed in the late stages of the disease. Most of the bursae show swollen bursal folds with ecchymotic to pinpoint haemorrhagic spots. Kidneys are swollen and show prominent uratic deposits in kidney tubules. Patchy haemorrhages on the mucosal surface at the junction of the gizzard and proventriculus are the most prominent lesions. Livers show fatty changes in most of the occasions.

Histopathological Lesions

Bursa of fabricious shows important microscopic findings, such as massive depletion of lymphoid cells and various stages of necrotic changes in bursal follicles, such as typical 'starry sky appearance', cystic degeneration and various stages of fibroplasias depending upon the stages of the disease. Heterophillic infiltrations and metaplasia of epithelium of bursal plicae are also seen.

In some instances, the hepatic parenchyma (liver) reveals various degenerative changes.

Control measures adopted

During the episode of VVIBD in India for the 1st time, various private sector hatchery groups and Agriculture/Veterinary universities and Govt. agencies from the country undertook a big task of bio-security and disinfection measures for bringing down the high levels of field virus load.

The ten point bio-security plan generally adopted by these groups to control the field virus was as follows:

1. Use of disinfectant foot baths/sprays at the entrance of farms (such as lime powder, formaldehyde, idophore compounds, gluteraldehyde based disinfectants, chloramines and quaternary ammonium compounds.
2. Proper cleaning and disinfection of sheds (flooring, walls, roofs, cages, feeders, waterers and brooders).
3. Proper disposal of poultry carcasses, used litter and used vaccine vials by burning.
4. Control of disease carrying vectors (ticks, mites, beetles, migratory birds and rats)
5. Discouraging multiple age groups on farms or at least in the same sheds.
6. Controlling access of men and materials on the farm.
7. Proper feeding, watering and routine dosing of coccidiostats, anti-bacterials, antihalmentics and avoiding stress due to debeaking, excessive handling of birds and water deprivation.
8. Use of potent vaccines and proper vaccination schedules.
9. Proper sanitation of drinking water and ample supply of clean and cool water.
10. Proper disinfection of incoming vehicles, egg trays and gunny bags of feed, etc.

The various hatchery groups in private sector also organized demonstration of disinfection, bio-security measures and vaccination programmes on some farms of opinion makers identified in various poultry belts. This could help in bringing down the incidence of VVIBD to a great extent in India by 1995-96. The credit of reduction in number of out breaks and severity of mortality pattern could be attributed to the increased awareness of farmers regarding bio-security and disinfection programmes adjuncted with proper vaccines and vaccination schedules and increased percentage of vaccination coverage. However, VVIBD still shows its prevalence and brings about high mortality upto 5% occasionally due to slackness in the bio-security/vaccination programme.

Vaccines, vaccination schedules and strategies

Prior to the striking of VVIBD in India during 1992, only IBD (Lukert) vaccine which is mildest of all vaccines was available on small scale and IBD (inactivated) oil adjuvanted vaccine was available only for breeder birds. This was responsible for large scale susceptibility of commercial flocks to VVIBD which results in catastrophic mortality of flocks in various poultry belts in India.

Later on IBD intermediate strain vaccines which have capacity to penetrate the moderate levels of maternal antibodies in chicks of 7-10 day age group, were permitted to be manufactured in India by 1994-95 by Govt. of India. These intermediate strain vaccines brought down the incidence of high mortality to moderate level mortality in VVIBD out breaks. However, introduction of hot strains of IBD vaccines from abroad, such as Intervet Bursin-2 and indigenous hot strains like Indovac IV-95 and later on Ventri's Intermediate Plus strains brought down the incidence of VVIBD to the satisfactory level as these hot invasive strains were able to penetrate very high levels of maternal immunity in the chicks in the age group of 15 to 20 days, when they needed the vaccine shot. However, these invasive vaccines were having capacity to produce immune-suppression of high to moderate levels and hence, their use, especially in the age groups of 7 to 12 days was desastrous. Hence, it was necessary to use these vaccines judiciously and vaccination schedules based on maternal immunity status of the flocks were found useful in effective control of VVIBD without much side effects/secondary complications. Use of Elisa Kits for study of maternal immunity was made by various hatchery groups successfully for designing of the vaccination schedule for VVIBD protection. Finding of 'window' in the maternal immunity of the chicks (titre below 1:500) was useful for advising the 'Vaccination day'.

Vaccination schedule

The following guidelines were useful in determining proper vaccination schedule for VVIBD:

1. If outbreaks are occurring cyclically during 3rd and 4th week period, use of 'mild lukert type' vaccine from 1st to 7th day, followed by use of 'Intermediate (standard) strain' on 12th to 14th day along with IBD inactivated vaccine simultaneously or alternatively use of only IBD intermediate plus vaccine on 14th day after priming with Lukert vaccine. IBD intermediate standard vaccine may be used for booster on 25th day, if outbreaks are occurring after 30 days.
2. If the outbreaks are occurring between 6th to 9th week with cyclical problems, use of IBD standard Intermediate strain + IBD (Inactivated) vaccine on 12th to 14th day or IBD Intermediate strain vaccine only on 12th to 14th day followed by repeat vaccination of IBD intermediate (standard) only on 22nd day followed by booster of the same on 30th day. Rarely there is a need of standard intermediate strain booster on 42nd day in case of outbreak on 9th week (Late IBD) is observed.
3. It is necessary to undertake IBD (inactivated) vaccination in layer/breeder flocks in pre-lay in layer/broiler breeder flocks in pre-lay period (16th -18th week) followed by mid-lay period (35-40 weeks) for conforming maternal immunity to the layer/broiler commercial progeny chicks for their protection in early use of 1 to 21 days on the commercial farms.

Suggested Reading

Chettle, N., Stuart, J.C. and Wyeth, P.J. (1989).Outbreak of virulent infectious bursal disease in East Anglia. Vet. Rec. 125: 271-272.

Cosgrove, A.S. (1962). An apparently new disease of chickens- avian nephrosis. Avian Dis. 6: 385-389.

Craft, D.W., Brown, J. and Lukert, P.D. (1990). Effects of standard and variant strains of infectious bursal disease virus on infections of chickens. Am J Vet Res. 51(8): 1192-7.

Ismail, N.M. and Saif, Y.M. (1991). Immunogenicity of infectious bursal disease viruses in chickens. Avian Dis. 35(3): 460-469.

Lukert, P.D. and. Saif, Y.M. (2003). Infectious bursal disease. In: Diseases of Poultry. 11th Ed., B.W. Calnek (ed.) Iowa State University Press, Ames, Iowa, USA. pp: 161-179.

Mc Ferran, J.B., Mc Nulty, M.S., Mc Killop, E.R., Connor, T.J., Mc Kracken, R.M., Collins, D.S. and Allen, G.M. (1980). Isolation and serological studies with infectious bursal disease viruses from fowl, turkeys and ducks; Demonstration of second serotype. Avian Pathol. 9: 395-403.

Mohanty, G.C., Pandey, A.P. and Rajya, B.S. (1971). Infectious bursal disease in chicken. Curr. Sci., 40: 181-184.

Nunoya, T., Otaki, Y.Tajima, M., Hiraga, M. and Saito, T. (1992). Occurrence of Acute Infectious Bursal Disease with High Mortality in Japan and Pathogenicity of Field Isolates in Specific-Pathogen-Free Chickens. Avian Diseases. 36(3): 597-609.

Report on Study group on poultry diseases – Infections Bursal Disease, Inclusion Body hepatitis and Avian influenza 'Appointed by Technology mission on dairy development' March, 1996.

Sah, R.L., Kataria, J.M., Arya, S.C. and Verma, K.C. (1995). Outbreak of acute infectious bursal disease causing high mortality in chicken. Indian J. Comp. Microbiol. Immunol. Infect. Dis., 16: 7-13.

Saif, Y.M., Jackwood, D.H., Jackwood, M.W. and Jackwood, D.J. (1987). Relatedness of IBD vaccine strains and field strains. Proceedings of the 36th Western Poultry Disease Conference, 110-111.

Saif, Y.M (2004). Control of infectious burial disease virus by vaccination. Dev. Biol. 119: 143-146.

Vandenberg, T.P., Gonze, M. and Meulemans, G. (1991). Acute infectious bursal disease in poultry: isolation and characterization of a highly virulent strain. Avian Pathol. 20: 133-143.

Very virulent infectious bursal disease (VVIBD) its prevention and control (1994). Booklet published by Institute of Poultry Management of India. (Wiley Eastern Limited, New Delhi, Bengaluru, Mumbai, Kolkata, Guwahati, Hyderabad, Lucknow, Chennai, Pune, London and new age International).

□□□

Chapter 5

Fowl Pox and Other Avian Poxes

Avian pox group of diseases have been reported in more than 60 species of wild and domestic birds representing 20 families. Avian pox group includes fowl pox which is a common viral disease of domestic birds including chicken turkeys, pigeons and canaries. Fowl pox is probably ancient most disease of birds. Fowl pox is a slow spreading viral disease characterized by the development of discreet nodular proliferative skin lesions on the non-feathered parts of the body. Cutaneous or fibrino-necrotic and proliferating lesions in the mucous membrane of upper respiratory tract, mouth and esophagus (Diphtheritic form) is called as cutaneous form and the later is called as diphtheritic form of the fowl pox. Avian pox has no public health significance. The disease is worldwide in distribution.

About the viruse(s)

Avian pox viruses (fowl, turkey, pigeon, canary, quail, sparrow, etc.) are belonging to 'Avipox virus' genus of the family *Poxviridae*. Fowl pox virus is the type species of the genus. Cross protection studies indicate pssitacine pox virus and myna pox virus are perhaps different members of the genus.

Avian pox viruses show identical morphology, thus mature virus (elementary body) is brick shaped with centrally located biconcave core (Nucleoid) and two lateral bodies in each concavity and envelop. The outer content is composed of randomly arranged tubules (Carter and Cheville, 1981).However, Dubochet *et al.* (1994) reported that fowl pox virus elementary body is brick shaped and is with uniform core and dumbbell shape core described previously was an artifact. Woodruff and Goodpasture (1931) described specific cellular cytoplasmic inclusion bodies of fowl pox virus (called as 'Bollinger bodies') which are composed of aggregates of elementary bodies (called as Borrel bodies) within the same (Bollinger body). The elementary bodies (Borrel bodies) were the etiological agent of fowl pox.

Fowl pox virus is a DNA virus with lot of lipid (mainly squalene) which constitutes nearly 1/3rd of the fowl pox virus. The viral genome is a single linear double stranded DNA molecule. Mathew (1982) reported that Fowl pox virus is resistant to ether which is one of the taxonomic criterions while according to Randall *et al.* (1964) Fowl pox virus is both ether and chloroform sensitive. Pigeon pox virus is resistant to both chloroform and ether. Fowl pox is known to withstand 1% Phenol and 1:1000 formaldehyde for 9 days but is inactivated by 1% caustic potash. It survives in dry scale for months or even years.

Fowl pox/pigeon pox viral DNA have similar genomic profiles while quail pox, canary pox and myna pox virus DNA revealed marked differences from fowl pox virus DNA. (Nazerian, *et al.*, 1989; Schnitzlein, *et al.*, 1988; Ghildyal, *et al.*, 1989) A nucleoprotein precipitinogen is common to all pox viruses (Woodroofe and Fenner, 1962) but avian pox viruses are antigenically and immunologically distinguishable from each other by complement fixation, passive haemalutination, agar gel diffusion precipitation, immune-peroxidase virus neutralization and immune fluorescence method with varying degrees of cross relationships.

Bird's susceptibility of different Avian Pox Viruses

Pox virus isolated from parrots was less pathogenic to chickens and did not provide protection against fowl pox virus in chickens (Boosinger, *et al.*, 1982). Vaccination of chickens with either fowl or pigeon pox virus vaccine did not provide protection against the psittacoses pox virus. Turkey pox virus isolates were antigenically different from fowl pox virus (Winterfield., *et al.*, 1985). Canaries are highly susceptible to canary pox virus but show resistance to turkeys, fowl and pigeon pox viruses. (Tripathy and Cunningham 1984). Similarly, pigeon pox virus produces severe disease in pigeons but produces only milder local pox lesions in poultry and turkeys (Hence, pigeon pox virus is used as vaccine virus strain for protection against fowl pox as both the viruses are closely related antigenically).

Susceptibility of developing chicken egg embryos

Most of the avian pox viruses from various avian species can grow and can be propogated on Choreo Allantoic Membrane (CAM) of chicken embryos (9 to 12 days old) which results into development of compact, proliferative pock lesions that may be focal or diffuse. Quantitative assay of viral infectivity may be by the embryo infective dose 50% (EID_{50}) method or by the 'Pock counting enumerative dose' response (Woodruff and Goodpasture, 1931; Cunningham, 1973).

Propagation of fowl pox virus on cell culture

Chicken embryo fibroblasts (CEF), chicken embryo dermis and chicken embryo kidney cells, duck embryo fibroblasts cell culture and Japanese quail permanent cell line 'QT 35' can be used for propagation of Avian pox viruses. 'QT 35' cell line may require serial passaging and adaptation of virus isolates.

Cytopathic effect (CPE) produced by avian pox viruses in CEF cultures is characterized by typical initial rounding of the cells which produces honey comb like appearance, followed by a second phase of degeneration, necrosis and coming out of cells in suspension of cell culture medium. Quantitative assay is by all the cell culture dose 50% method based on CPE.

Avian pox viruses after adaptation to cell cultures have ability to produce plaques in most but not all cases. Some of the avian pox virus plaques have specific characteristics which can differentiate from each other.

Pathogenesis and Epizootology

In chicken infected intradermally, the virus is first detected in the skin at the inoculation site on 2nd day followed by in lungs on 4th day and detectable viremia on day 5th while in chickens infected by intra-tracheal route, virus in found in lungs on 2nd day and viremia on 4th day. It can be recovered from spleen, liver, kidneys and brain in both the groups. Incubation period of fowl pox virus is estimated to be from 4 to 10 days in nature.

In nature, infection occurs through mechanical transmission of the virus to the injured or lacerated skin. The virus can be spread by the workers in the poultry sheds through their hands or cloathings. Mosquitoes, flies and mites can also act as mechanical spreaders of the disease.

In contaminated environment, the aerosol generated by feathers and dried scabs containing virus particles provides suitable environment for both cutaneous and respiratory infection.

Once fed singly on infected bird, mosquitoes are capable to infect number of susceptible birds in the flocks in the same shed or adjacent sheds by bite mechanically. Similar transmission is possible through mites belonging to the species Dermanyss gallinae and the flies (Diptera) of 11 species.

Mechanical transmission through artificial insemination is also reported in case of turkey hens due to infected farms (Metry, *et al.*, 1985).

Recently, pox virus have been isolated in mid west, south east and north-west United States from previously standard Fowl pox vaccinated flocks, showing both diphtheritic and cutaneous pox. Cross protection tests revealed that these pox strains were not having serological relationships or immunological relationship with standard fowl pox virus used in fowl pox vaccines but they were closely related with pigeon pox vaccine strain (Reed, *et al.*, 1994).

Symptoms

Generally, disease occurs in 2 forms namely cutaneous form and diptheritic from separately. However, both the forms can be observed in single outbreak also.

Cutaneous form is characterized by nodular lesions on the comb, wattles, eyelids and other non feathered parts of the body.

Cankers or yellowish diphtheritic lesions on the mucous surface of the mouth oesophagus or trachea with coryza like symptoms are seen in 'Wet pox' (diphtheritic form) disease.

Morbidity varies between 1% to even upto 60-70% and mortality in cutaneous form may be negligible while it can go from 1 to 5% or even upto 50-60% in case of diphtheritic form depending upon stress factors or immune suppression due to IBD or CAA infection concurrently.

Blindness can occur due to cutaneous eye lesions and death due to starvation in such birds. Decreased egg production is the major cause of economic loss in cutaneous fowl pox.

Canary pox can cause even 100% mortality in aviaries and quail pox results into heavy losses (deaths) in quailaries.

Gross lesions & Histopathology

Characteristic lesion of cutaneous pox is local epithelial hyperplasia in dermis and under lying feather follicles, with formation of nodules, first appearing as while foci, rapidly increasing in size and becoming yellow. Primary lesion appears by 4th day of infection followed by Papule (Yellow) formation on 5th to 6th day. This is followed by vesicle formation with extensive thick lesion. Lesions adjoining each other coalesce become rough and grey or dark brown. By 2nd week or earlier lesion's base becomes haemorrhagic or inflamed. Scale formation lasts for 1-2 weeks further, which when removed in early stage, shows moist sero-purulent exudates, covering a haemorrhagic granulating surface. If scale falls after natural course, a smooth scar remains.

In diphtheritic form, while opaque nodule develop on mucous membrane which rapidly coalesce to become a yellow, cheesy, necrotic diphtheritic membrane. These when removed, leave bleeding erosions. These lesion's may be observed even extended upto infra orbital sinus which may result into coryza like swelling. Such lesion in pharynx and larynx and esophagus may result into respiratory disturbances.

The histopathological picture of the pox lesion on dermis, mucous membrane and/or CAM of infected embryo is characterized by hyperplasia of epithelium with associated inflammatory reaction. Epithelial cells affected by pox virus show typical 'intracytoplasmic' 'type A' inclusion bodies (Bollinger bodies) which stain pink by Haematoxalin-eosion stain. Clusters of epithelial cells resemble like papilloma. The inclusions may occupy entire cytoplasm which results in cell necroses.

Diagnostic tests

Typical cutaneous nodular lesions described above are quite diagnostic of fowl pox clinically. However, presence of the cytoplasmic inclusions and typical histo-pathological picture in the cutaneous/ mucous membrane lesions after H.E. staining described under the histo-pathology is quite diagnostic of fowl pox.

This clinical diagnosis of fowl pox can be further confirmed by virus isolation on CAM of 9-11 days old susceptible egg embryos (SPF origin) and further serological confirmation by AGPT is sufficient for fowl pox diagnosis.

Electron microscopy can be employed for demonstration of virus particles (elementary bodies - Borrel bodies) in cytoplasmic inclusions (Bollinger bodies) in infected cells or in exudates by negative staining or in ultra thin sections of infected tissues (Mc. Ferran *et al.*, 1971 and Van Kammen and Spadbrow, 1976).

Immunity and Serology

Cell mediated and humoral immunity following vaccination or naturally occurring infection brings about protection against fowl pox infection.

Protection tests are generally employed to determine immunogenicity of fowl pox and pigeon pox vaccines.

Cross protection tests for the antigenic relationships of the avian pox viruses are practiced for characterization of their antigens. (Winterfield, *et al.*, 1985).

Agar gel immuno diffusion precipitation test (AGPT)

It is performed on sera usually collected 15-20 days post infection for differential identification of fowl pox, pigeon pox and other avian pox viral infections (Jordan and Chubb, 1962; Uppal and Nilkantan, 1970). Passive haemagglutination (Chung *et al.*, 1977), Neutralisation (Baxendale, 1971), FAT and ELISA (Buscaglia, *et al.*, 1985 and Mockett, *et al.*, 1987) are other diagnostic tests used by some workers. Immunoblotting used to detect common sharing antigens between fowl pox and vaccinia virus.

Preventive Vaccines

Two types of live attenuated fowl pox vaccines are available for protection of chickens. Fowl pox vaccine produced on CAM of SPF egg embryos in freeze dried form is the most commonly used vaccine for protection against fowl pox in the field. It being produced on chick embryo itself, it is supposed to be highly immunogenic and it has the titre of at least 10^5 ID_{50}/ml for establishing satisfactory 'takes' to produce good immunity. The vaccine is glycernised and hence, vaccine sticks to lacerated skin surface properly to produce good take. This vaccine can be applied to the birds above 6-8 weeks of age and hence, it is unsuitable for use before 6 weeks of age in young chicks. It is highly pathogenic for young chickens.

Fowl fox virus of CAM origin is further attenuated and adapted to grow in chick embryo fibroblast cultures of SPF origin (CEF culture origin vaccine virus). This virus is used for vaccination of chicks below 6 weeks of age.

Pigeon pox virus is highly antigenically related to fowl pox virus but pigeon pox virus is not pathogenic much to the chickens and hence, pigeon pox vaccine virus grown on CAM or CEF of SPF chick origin can be safely used for vaccination of chicks below 6 weeks of age or even in chicks above 6 weeks to 18 weeks of age.

Prophylactic vaccination against fowl pox is indicated under 3 conditions:

1. When flock on the premises is infected, the previous year with fowl pox and all young stock produced on the premises or introduced from other sources should receive fowl pox vaccine.
2. If pox was present the previous year, when 'pigeon fox vaccine' was used birds should be re-vaccinated with 'Fowl pox vaccine' as pigeon pox vaccine immunity is not of long duration.
3. In areas where pox is prevalent, fowl pox vaccine should be used for protection against infection from the neighboring flocks.

Fowl pox scenario in India

As described earlier in columns on New castle disease, fowl pox and ND were the only significant two diseases of poultry in India up-to early nineteen sixties. IVRI, Izatnagar (Biological Products Division) and State Veterinary Biological Products Divisions were producing effective fowl pox vaccine for use in grower birds after 8 weeks of age and that kept the disease under control during those days. However, due to the expanding poultry industry during nineteen sixties and seventies and presence of the multiple age group poultry farms increasing with poor bio-security and disinfection conditions, age groups of chicks lower than 8 weeks of age started getting exposed to fowl pox resulting into clinical fowl pox precipitation. Pigeon pox vaccine strain being milder for the poultry birds, IVPM Ranipet in late nineteen sixties started producing pigeon pox vaccine which proved useful for vaccination of chicks as early as 3-4 weeks age and thus could protect younger chicks from the disease.

Cell culture origin vaccine for chickens above 6 weeks of age was used in early nineteen eighties, when IBD and CAA subclinical infections brought about immune suppression problems which brought above problems of precipitation of fowl pox in age group below 6 weeks of age (3 weeks onwards), with manifestations of naso-pharyngeal diphtheritic form of the disease with high mortality, in spite of standard fowl pox vaccination, experimental vaccine using pigeon pox vaccine virus or cell culture adapted vaccine virus of fowl pox suitably modified for use in one day old chicks was used with some success for two weeks early age chick vaccination especially in south.

During late nineteen nineties and early two thousand one onwards, pox infections probably belonging to other avian pox groups started producing 'Pox' of diphtheritic or cutaneous pox with higher mortalities. Pigeon pox vaccine proved useful in such problems in north.

Suggested Reading

Buscaglia, C.,Bankowaski, R.A. and Miers, L. (1985). Cell-culture virus-neutralization test and enzyme-linked immunosorbent assay for evaluation of immunity in chickens against fowlpox. Avian Dis. 29(3): 672-80.

Bxendale, W. (1971). Studies of three avian pox virusesand development of an improved fowlpox vaccine. Vet. Rec 88(1).5-10. Cunningham; C.H. (1973). A Laboratory Guide in Virology, 7th Edition. Burgess Publishing Co.

Boosinger, T.R., Winterfield, R.W., Feldman, D.S. and Dhillon, A.S. (1982). Psittacine pox virus: virus isolation and identification, transmission, and cross-challenge studies in parrots and chickens. Avian Dis.; 26(2): 437-44.

Carter, J.K. and Cheville N.F. (1981). Isolation of surface tubules of fowl pox virus. Avian Dis. 25(2): 454-462.

Dubochet, J., Adrian, M., Richter, K., Garces, J., Wittek, R. (1994). Structure of intracellular mature vaccinia virus observed by cryoelectron microscopy, J. Virol. 68: 1935-1941.

Ghildyal, M.N., Schnitzlein, W.N. and Tripathy, D.N. (1989). Genetic and antigenic differences between fowlpox and quailpox viruses. Archives of Virology 106: 85–92.

Jordan, F.T.W. and Chubb, R.C. (1962). The agar gel diffusion technique in the diagnosis of infectious laryngo-tracheitis (I.L.T.) and its differentiation from fowl pox. Res. Vet. Sci. 3: 245-255.

Mc Ferran, I.B., Clorke, J.K. and Curran, W.L. (1971). The application of negative contrast elecctron microscopy to routine veterinary virus diagnosis. Res.Vet. Sci 12: 253-257.

Mathew, R.E.F. (1982). Classification and nomenclature of viruses. Intervirology. 17: 42-46.

Mockett, A.P.A., Southee, D.J., Tomley, F.M. and Deuter, A. (1987). Fowlpox virus: its structural proteins and immunogens and the detection of viral-specific antibodies by ELISA. Avian Pathology, 16: 493-504.

Nazerian, K.S., Dhawale, S. and Payne, W.S. (1989). Structural proteins of two different plaque size phenotypes of fowlpox virus. Avian Dis. 33: 458-465.

Randall, C.C., Gafford, L.G., Darlington, R.W. and Hyde, J. (1964). Composition of fowlpox virus and matrix.J. Bacteriol. 87: 939-944.

Schnitzlein, W.N., Ghildyal, M.N. and Tripathy, D.N. (1988). Genomic and antigenic characterization of avipoxviruses. Virus Research 10: 65–76.

Tripathy, D.M. and Cunningham, C.H. (1984). Avian pox. In: Diseases of Poultry, 8th edition, pp. 524-534. Edited by Hofstad, M.S., John Barnes, H., Calnek, B.W., Reid, W.M. and Yoder, H.W. Ames, Iowa: Iowa State University Press.

Uppal, P.K. and Nilakantan, P.R. (1970). Studies on the serological relationships between avian pox, sheep pox, goat pox and vaccinia viruses. Journal of Hygiene. 68(3): 349-58.

Van Kammen, A. and Spadbrow, P.B. (1976). Rapid diagnosis of some avian virus diseases. Avian Dis., 20: 748–751.

Woodruff, G.M. and Goodpasture (1931). The susceptibility of chorio-allantoic membrane of chick embryos to infection with fowl pox virus. Am. J. Pathol. 7(3): 209-222.

Woodruff, G.M. and Fenner, F. (1962). Serological relationships within pox virus group: an antigen common to all members of the group. Virology, 16: 334-341.

❑❑❑

Chapter 6

Marek's Disease: Ever Changing Strategies of Vaccination and Control – Indian Scenario

Marek's Disease (MD) is an important neoplastic disease of chickens, first recognized during 1907. This disease causes tumours, detrimental effect on production and mortality. Unlike Lymphod Leucosis another tumour forming avian disease is also known as Avian Leucosis Complex (ALC). It is not transmitted vertically. Only horizontal transmission of the disease through shading of MD virus in the feather follicle's epithetical cells (Dander) in the affected house occurs. This is important source of infection from older flocks to new replacements. The house dust containing virus remains infective for months together on the farm environment. The MD vaccines protect the birds against the disease (Tumour formation) but not against the infection with virus upon exposure in the field.

About the MD virus

Marek's disease virus is classified under *Herpesviridae* family. Based on neutralization test and AGPT analysis, 3 antigenically related serotypes of the virus are recognized:

1. MDV serotype-1 : Pathogenic and attenuated strains.
2. MDV serotype-2 : Non-onchogenic strains
3. Turkey Herpes Virus (HVT) : Non pathogenic naturally occurring strain

Serotype-3

Based on pathogenecity, the serotype 1 MDV strains are further differentiated in 4 'Pathotypes' as described below. These pathotypes are evolved in the field over the time due to the natural mutation in the 'Virulence genes' of the field virus on account of 'Vaccination pressure' created by the commercial breeders using newer and higher grade vaccines in the birds (Witter, 1996).

These pathotypes are as follows:

- M – MDV : Mild MDV
- V – MDV : Virulent MDV
- VV-MDV : Very Virulent MDV
- VV + - MDV : Very Virulent plus MDV (Hyper virulent hv)

Stepwise Evolution of Virulent MDV Isolates

Moderate MDV causes neural lesions and virulent MDV also causes neural lesions but of more severe nature. However, VV-MDV causes lymphomas in visceral organs even in 6 weeks aged chickens while VV + MDV bring about 'transient paralysis' in 2-3 weeks old chickens due to brain involvement. It is also capable of transmission of lymphomas in adult vaccinated and immune competent birds with high infectivity (Late Marek's Disease).

Transmission of Marek's Disease Virus

The field MD virus is contained in skin cells/feather follicles of infected bird. The sloughing of old skin and feather follicle cells contain MD virus which is carried in air along with the dust in chicken houses. The susceptible chickens breathe in these dust particles along with the virus particles. The virus particles are carried through blood circulation to bursa of fabricious of the birds, wherein first multiplication of the virus occurs followed by viremia and ultimate multiplication of the virus in visceral organs and finally in the skin cells/feather follicle epithelium. This takes 2 weeks which is the minimum time taken to become bird as potential shedder of the virus. Bird need not die and even the normal MD vaccinated otherwise healthy bird can also become shedder and carrier of the virus.

Vaccination and control measures

Following the introduction of MD HVT FC-126 vaccine during 1971 for the first time in the world, there was dramatic reduction in losses in broiler and layer birds. However, the evolution and shift in pathotypes mentioned previously, over the time resulted in a potential for greater disease losses that was persistent until more effective vaccination was introduced. The condition that favours evolution are obscure but may be due to compromise of the vaccine immunity by early exposure or the immune suppressive stress increase the opportunity of mutant clones to selectively multiply in vaccinated flocks. There is a race between the vaccine virus producing immunity and field virus exposure initiating productive infection in the chicks.

About the MD vaccines

Presently individual and combination of MD vaccines are available for control of MDV all over the world.

Sr. No.	Vaccines	Serotypes
1.	FC-126 HVT, live freeze dried	Serotype-3
2.	FC-126 HVT, live cell Associated and combinations	Serotype-3
3.	SB-1/301 B cell - Associated and combinations	Serotype-2
4.	Rispens (CVI 988) cell - Associated and other attenuated strains And combinations	Serotype-1

The efficacy of MD vaccines to control MD pathogens is graded as below. Efficacy of vaccines V/S pathotypes.

Pathotypes

Sr. No.	Vaccines	M/V MDV	VV MDV	VV + MDV
1.	HVT	+++	+	+
2.	Bivalent (HVT + SB1)	+++	+++	++
3.	Rispens (CVI - 988)	+++	+++	+++

Monovalent vaccine has shown its efficacy but combination of one or more strains of MD vaccine has shown protective synergism for better protection. HVT + SB1 bivalent vaccine has proved best in present situation of VVMDV with field exception. It needs more investigation to characterize the present pathotypes causing such breaks and other possible causes including immune suppression in the field due to CAA, IBDV, Reo viruses.

Review of Marek's Disease – Indian Scenario

Marek's Disease first showed its existence in India in early nineteen sixties of 20th century especially around 1965. It produced number of outbreaks in commercial layer farms, with the prominent symptom of 'neural paralyses', including typical posture of 'one leg forward and one leg backward'. This produced panic in breeders of Bombay-Pune belt as no preventive vaccination and the curative treatment was available for this malady during those days in India. Some breeders like 'Hyline Poultry brooding Farm' Aundh (Pune) were closed down due to this situation around 1974-75.

Some breeders like 'Arbor Acres' in Bombay-Pune belt imported Marek's HVT FC-126 freeze dried vaccine from abroad to cope up with the havoc created by Marek's Disease around 1975-76. The BAIF (Bharatiya Agro Industries Foundation) Uruli Kanchan, District Pune launched Adhoc scheme for Research of Marek's disease with special reference to development of suitable vaccine on 1st October, 1976, which lasted upto September, 1981.

Dr. B.V. Rao of Venkateshwara Hatcheries, with the experience of previous Marek's Disease Problem at 'Arbor Acres, Talagaon, Distt. Pune' floated the idea of production of Marek's disease vaccine in India during the same period (1976 to 1980) and was able to produce Marek's Disease vaccine under the collaboration of Tri-Bio, Laboratory, State College Pensylvania, USA, in1980 at Ventri Biologicals Division of his own Venkateshwara Hatcheries Ltd., Pune. Ventri Biological's Marek's Disease Vaccine, HVT (FC-126 strain), living, Freeze Dried, took care of Poultry Industry in India against the incidences of Marek's Disease very effectively for the period of 6 to 7 years upto about 1987, when slowly the Marek's Disease 'Breaks' started occurring in Vaccinated flocks. We took care of these 'breaks' by introduction of practice of Booster Marek's Disease vaccination at 'Farm level' 21 days after the initial MD vaccination at one day age at 'Hatchery level', presuming that there can be some vaccination 'slips' in the chicks during mass one day age MD vaccination at hatchery level. It was also presumed that good number of chicks may be possessing higher maternal antibody levels in them due to vaccination followed by exposure to the field infection in the parent birds which might have caused hyperimmune antibody situation in parent birds, resulting into higher maternal Antibody status in the commercial chicks. Thus, day old hatchery level MD vaccination must be neutralizing the MD vaccine virus, resulting into failure of hatchery level MD vaccination. The Booster MD vaccination is carried out on 21st day of age at commercial farm level in those chicks with high 'MAB status' with the idea that the higher 'MAB' is 'waning' by 21st day and 'window' for entry of 'Booster' vaccine virus is made available for successful 'Vaccine take'. The 'Booster Vaccination' concept was most successful in India, even though the explanation given by us was not well accepted by the scientists from abroad (especially U.S. Scientists), we could very effectively stop the Marek's Disease 'breaks' in India by use of 'Booster" M.D. Vaccination. Thus, there was 'Lull' on 'Marek's' disease front in India upto 1994 at breeder and commercial farm levels.

During 1996 onwards, large scale 'MD' outbreaks were observed in Hyderabad and Mysore layer belts. The investigation revealed that the use of Hot IBD vaccines brought about immune suppression in chicks at early age which resulted into poor immunological responses to MD vaccinations. The farmers were enlightened by Ventri-Bio-PDRC scientists on this issue. They were advised to purchase one day old commercial chicks only from specified parent hatcheries, wherein we undertook Cell Associated HVT + SB1 (Cell Associated) Bivalent Vaccination in breeder chicks (one day old) which then resulted in parent flock with high levels of antibodies against Marek's Disease. This resulted in commercial chicks (one day old) from our hatcheries with high levels of 'maternal MD antibodies' i.e. passive antibodies in them inspite of exposure of these chicks to IBD virus during the 1st 21 days and thus, could not produce active MD immunity by 'day old' hatchery level MD vaccination. These passive MD antibodies could protect these chicks from field MD virus exposure during 1st 21 days. The farmers were also advised not to use hot IBD virus for protection of their chicks against IBD, but to use IBD standard Intermediate vaccine along with IBD (in activated) vaccine for proper IBD protection without immune suppression. They were also advised to undertake Booster MD vaccination on 6th to 15th days at farm level instead of carrying out the same on 18th to 21st day. This could have protected the commercial chicks which are now not immune suppressed due to hot vaccine usages as was being done previously. This 'complicated strategy' of use of:

1. HVT FC-126 + SB1, cell Associated vaccine in parent breeder chicks at hatchery level.

2. IBD standard intermediate vaccine + IBD (inactivated) vaccine in the commercial chicks at 7-10 days age without using only HOT IBD vaccine in them and.
3. Booster MD (HVT-C-126 F.D.) vaccine in these commercial chicks at 6th to 15th day age instead of using the same on 18th to 21st day was found rewarding and we could successfully came out of MD problems in that area within 4 months time.

During October, 1997, large scale 'MD vaccination outbreaks' were reported in the integrators Broiler breeding 'parent' flocks at Jind and Gurgaon originating from their great grandparent stock in October, 1996. The reason was traced out as poor quality parent chicks in which sufficient maternal Antibodies (MAB) against MD were not transferred by their ground grandparent chicks, resulting into low MAB titres which receded faster and hence, they became 'prone' to the field MD exposure before 'booster vaccination' at integrator farm level which was carried out on 18th day. Moreover, it was also suspected that the 'handling' of cell Associated HVT + SB1 vaccine reconstitution might not have been done properly for want of sufficient training of vaccinators at Hatchery level.

During the period of November, 1998 to December, 1998, 'Sangrur (Punjab)' commercial lager belt along with Barwala layer belt was badly affected with Marek's disease problem. Moreover, M.D. outbreaks were also reported from larger number of Broiler breeders in Jind (Haryana) and Gurgaon belts. Wide scale Marek's Disease problems were also noticed in Kashipur (U.P.) layer poultry belt. All the above outbreaks were from Punjab, Haryana and U.P. which were showing one common characteristic that thymus, bursa and spleens were showing typical atrophic changes with depletion of lymphocytes suggestive of severe immune suppression, which is either characteristic of VVMD + strains described by Calnec et al or possibility of accompaniment of Chicken Anaemia Agent (CAA) infection along with VVMD. The later possibility was more and it was further confirmed serologically and Histo-pathologically. It was, therefore, decided to have three pronged attack on this Marek's Disease Problems, namely:

1. Use of cell Associated HVT (FC-126) strain + SB1, strain vaccine at Hatchery level (in one day old chicks).

2. Monitoring of storage of cell Associated MD vaccines and their reconstitution at hatchery level, including through training of vaccinators.

3. Use of Booster HVT (FC-126) Freeze dried vaccination at earlier age between 10 to 15 days instead of 18 to 20 days.

This production of HVT and SBI cell Associated vaccines which was started at Ventri Biologicals Laboratory since 1994-95, was further boosted up from 1999-2000, as more and more breeder farms started using cell Associated Bivalent vaccination progrmames. This strategy paid rich dividends in the form of effective control of Marek's Disease Problems in previously highly affected areas like Mysore, Hyderabad, Haryana, Punjab and U.P. since year 2000-2001.

The Marke's Disease situation in the 'parent' and 'grandparent' flocks in the country was so much worsened due to prevalence of Chicken Anaemia Agent (CAA) infection that these breeder flocks especially in Punjab, Haryana and Hyderabad regions started showing clinical symptoms of CAA in breeder grower birds, even after the classically known CAA susceptibility age of 6 weeks is over. This was followed by incidence of Marek's Disease (clinical) in these parent and grandparent stocks. This resulted in very high levels of MD maternal antibodies in their commercial chicks. This very high levels of MAB were not receding even upto 21 days age of the commercial chicks. This brought about neutralization of MD vaccine virus in the Marek's Disease vaccines used for immunization of one day old commercial chicks which resulted into failure of one day old M.D. Vaccination at commercial hatchery level as well as failure of booster vaccinations which were being done at 6 to 15 days since 2001 as described previously. This all episode resulted into failure of Marek's Disease vaccination (primary and booster) in commercial layer and Broiler breeder parents in these poultry belts during the year 2005 to 2006 and Large scale M.D. outbreaks were found being precipitated in those poultry belts.

The strategy to undertake: 1) Vaccination of one day old parent/ chicken commercial with killed (inactivated) CAA vaccination by suitable route, followed by MD (Cell Associated) Bivalent vaccination (6 hours after CAA killed vaccination), 2) Booster Cell Associated MD bivalent vaccination of these parent/commercial chicks after 18 to 21 days (after monitoring of MAB status), was having limited success. It was also suspected that commercial MD vaccines do not contain adequately high levels of MD vaccine virus titres and hence, to take reviews of the commercial vaccine titres and their improvements were suggested by the consultants for improving the deteriorated MD outbreak situation in the country.

Genetics : No commercial layer variety is completely resistant to MD. However, selection can be done to gradually improve resistance. Of course this needs to be kept in balance with genetic selection for the other commercially valuable traits. It has been shown that vaccines will work better in the more genetically resistant lines. It is probably also time that ever improving vaccines may not be available to control future MD problems. The breeder industry must take responsibility to provide more genetically resistant varieties. 'Hyline' breeders are trying to select such resistant varieties for about a quarter of a century. They discovered certain 'blood types' in birds with genetic M.D. resistance. The new techniques of molecular biology are now being used which may provide a way to more quickly develop a M.D. resistant line.

Further strategies : MD being an evolving pathogen, it is extremely unlikely that MD will ever be completely eliminated from chicken population. We can only hope to design any effective strategy to control MD. We will have to evolve 'multiple approach' in face of evolution of MD pathotypes. The multiple approaches may include:

1. Developing new effective vaccines using rDNA technology with Fowl Pox virus vector expressing of B gene of MDV for vaccine production.
2. Breeding lines of chickens resistant to MD: Development of chickens with multiple lost resistant genes of 'MHC types'. The recent research work on genomic mapping of chickens to identify gene responsible for Non-MHC associated resistance in chickens is reported to be encouraging.
3. The breeding programme to express transcend in germ lines or somatic cells to limit the expression of MD challenge virus is another way out in MD control.
4. Better management practices like 'All in – all out' to prevent exposures of next young generation on the farm. Use of 'Filtered Air housing system' applied for SPF flock may only be practicable for breeding of 'important lines' against emerging virulent pathogens.

5. Control of immune suppressive diseases and stress factors to reduce MD problems.

Overall, it may be concluded that only vaccination will not work and the combination of all the above approaches religiously may control the problem.

Suggested Reading

Witter, R.L. (1996). Evolution of virulence of Marek's disease virus: evidence for a novel pathotype. In R.F. Silva, H.H. Cheng, P.M. Coussens, L.F. Lee & L.F. Velicer (Eds) Current Research on Marek's Disease (pp. 86-91). Kennett Square: American Association of Avian Pathologists.

□□□

Chapter 7

Avian Leukosis / Sarcoma Group of Diseases

Avian Leukosis/Sarcoma group of diseases consists of a number of neoplastic disease conditions of poultry caused by viruses of the family *Retroviridae*. These avian retroviruses are presently termed as 'avian leucosis virus (ALV)' which are characterized by similar physical and molecular characteristics, sharing a common group specific antigen.

Chubb and Gardon (1957) in their review on the avian leukosis complex have quoted the oldest occurrence of 'Lymphosarcomata' recorded by Roloff in 1868 and caprini described Lymphoid Leukemia in 1896. Butterfield described 'aleukemic Lymphadenosis' in USA in 1905 and alderman recorded 'Leucosis of fowl' in UK, in 1921. Biggs (1961) coined the term 'Avian Leukosis complex' and differentiated it from 'Fowl Paralysis' i.e. Marek's Disease (Biggs and Payne, 1964). Furth (1933) indicated filterability of lymphoid leukosis tumour producing agent which was proven ultimately with proof by Burmester, *et al.* (1947).

Ellermann and Bang (1908) reported experimental transmission of Erythroblastosis and viral etiology of the same was established by Burmester, *et.al.* (1959). Erythroblastosis and myeloblostosis were produced by 'BAT-A' virus strain but passages carried out with selection and cleaning of this virus strain resulted into variety of tumors. Fibro-sarcomas and mayo-sarcomas were first transmitted by free filtrates by Rous-sarcoma virus in 1911. Leukosis viruses were shown to cause other epithelial tumors including hepatcarcinomas (Lapis, 1979).

Incidence of Disease

Lymphoid Leukosis and related group of viruses produce infection in almost all chicken flocks with only few exceptions but the clinical disease is manifested in very low number of birds in general.

Occasionally, lymphoid leucosis (LL) can produce heavy looses in commercial breeders flocks. DeBoer, *et al.* (1981) reported 2.18 per cent L.L. in white layer's mortality in Netherlands, while 0.57 per cent mortality in brown layers.

Erythroblastosis occurs very infrequently under field conditions are compared to LL incidences. Myeloblastosis occurrence is 'sporadic' in nature. Similarly, mylo-cytomatosis occur sporadically. However, an overall incidence of 27 per cent mylo-cytomatosis was reported in broiler chickens inoculated with strain HPRS-103 of sub groups J ALV (Payne, *et al.*, 1992).

Of all tumours other than leukotic tumours, haemangiomas make upto 25 per cent and nephroblastomas 19 per cent in broilers and 19 per cent haemangiomas and 3-10 per cent Nephroblastomas in layers respectively (Cambell J.G. 1966 & Purchase H.G. *et al.*, 1972). Incidence of connective tissue tumour (sarcomas) in chickens is less than 1 in 1000 but epizootics are also recorded (Purchase H.G. *et al.*, 1972).

Osteopetrosis occurs widely, but much less frequently than L.L. Males are more frequently affected than female with Osteopetrosis.

About the virus(es)

Viruses of the Leukosis/sarcoma group belong to a genus termed provisionally as ALV related virus of the family *'Retroviridae'*. These RNA viruses possess the enzyme 'Reverse transcriptase' which is necessary for formation of a DNA 'Provirus' during viral replication.

The viruses of Leukosis/Sarcoma group are closely related and they cause a variety of neoplasms. These viruses are divided into 6 sub-groups, namely A,B,C,D and J on the basis of their host range in chicken embryo fibroblasts of different genetic types, interference pattern with members of the same and different sub-groups and viral envelop antigens identified by virus serum neutralization tests (Weiss R.A. *et al.*, 1982). These various properties are a reflection of the 'envelop glycoprotein's' present on the virus.

Sub-group A and B viruses are common exogenous viruses occurring in chickens in the field (Cinke, B.W. 1968) while sub-groups C and D viruses only rarely reported in the field (Morgen, H.R. 1973 and Sandelin, K. *et al.*, 1974). Sub groups E viruses are the ubiquitous Endogenous leukosis viruses of low Pathogenecity (Smith, E.H. 1987). The normal chicken cellular genome contains several classes or families of avian retrovirus like elements including endogenous viral (e.v.) loci. These genetic sequences of the e.v. loci are related to sub-groups E ALVs and are present as either complete or defective genomes in almost all normal chickens (Critenden, L.B. 1981). These e.v. loci have been located on particular chromosomes, occur in somatic and germ line cells and are transmitted genetically in 'Mendelian fashion' to their progeny by both sexes (Crittenden, *et al.*, 1977).

Viruses of sub-groups F and G are found in Ring necked pheasants while sub-group H are endogenus viruses found in Hungerian partyridges and sub-group I is present in gambel quail. (Figure *et al.*, 1974) sub-group J viruses were isolated recently from meat type chicken (Payne, L.N. *et al.*, 1992).

The viruses of all the sub groups cause a variety of neoplasms with 'short' to 'long' period of 'clinical latencies' depending upon their 'genetic make-up'. Mainly some 'laboratory propogated' strains, such as Avian sarcoma viruses (ASV) belonging to sub-groups A,B,C,D and E (Rous sarcoma viruses A,B,C,D and E i.e. RSVS) Avian erythroblastosis virus (AEV) with no sub-group and Avian myeloblastosis virus (AMV) with no sub-group cause 'rapid' development of tumours after quick neoplastic transformation within few days or weeks due to the fact that they carry specific 'Viral oncongenes' (called as 'V-one' genes) while other 'field isolates' of ALVS from 'lymphoid leukasis' cases cause transformation and tumour development very slowly, as they lack such viral oncogens (V oncogenes). These L.L. viruses take many weeks or many months for production of 'Clinical Tumours' after inoculation of the virus(es) in the chicken. This happens due to the fact that these viruses have to take help of 'Cellular' genes (proto-oncogens), such as 'C-myc' genes present on cellular genome as they themselves lack V-oncogens required for transformation and tumor formation in the host bird (Cooper, G.M. 1982).

Virus replication

The retrovirus ALV replication cycle has 4 steps, namely: 1) Attachment and Penetration of the host cell, 2) Synthesis and integration of viral DNA, 3) Formation of new virions in the infected cell as a result of 'transcription' and 'translation' of 'Pro-viral DNA', 4) Cell 'transformation' and tumor formation through V-onc (viral oncogens) or C-myc (culture oncogens) integration of 'Pro viral DNA'. These steps of virus replication are elaborated as follows:

1. **Penetration of Host cell :** Adsorption of virion to the cell membrane is non-specific but penetration of host cell is depending upon the occurrence of host gene encoded receptors specific for each virus sub-group. Dales and Hanafusa (1972) observed that virions are taken in the cell vacuoles and viral RNA in the nucleus within 120 minutes post attachment on cell surface receptors.
2. **Synthesis and integration of proviral DNA :** The unique feature of avian RNA retrovirus characteristics during viral replication is the formation of retroviral DNA (Provirus) from a template of viral RNA under the influence of viral 'Reverse transcriptase' enzyme of its own. This 'DNA Provirus' gets integrated into the host cell genome. Formation of new viral RNA takes place from the proviral DNA template. This process occurs in 4 stages as follows:
   i) Synthesis of the 1st (minus) strand of viral DNA, forming an RNA: DNA hybrid.
   ii) Removal of RNA from hybrid by R Nase-4 enzyme and formation of second (plus) standards of viral DNA on the template of minus strand DNA giving rise to liniar DNA duplexes which are detectable in cell cytoplasm within few hours of infection.
   iii) Migration of linear DNA to cell nucleus.
   iv) Integration of linear viral DNA into the Host DNA in the nucleus under the influence to enzyme 'Integrase', which occurs at many sites and thus, infected cell nucleus may contain up to 20 copies of viral DNA in this way. The proviral genes occur in the same order as their RNA copies occur in the virion and they are flanked on either side by identical sequences of Nucleotides long terminal repeats (LTRS). These are composed of repeated sequences derived from terminal regions of viral RNA and include promoter and enhancer sequences controlling transcription of viral DNA to RNA. The LTR promoters may also cause abnormal transcription of host genes usually downstream of the proviral DNA leading to oncogenesis.
3. **Transcription :** 'Transcription' and 'Translation' of proviral DNA results into formation of new virions as follows:
   i) Hosts RNA polymerase brings about the transcription of viral RNA on a template of proviral DNA. Viral RNA molecules

give rise to m RNA (messenger RNA) in association of polyribosomes (which also serve as genomic RNA in the newly formed virions). New viral RNA is detected within 24 hours after infection.

ii) m RNA bound to polyribosomes are translated to form the gag, pol and e nv gene coded proteins that compose the virion. The gag-pol gene product is a large protein precursor which is cleaved to give rise to a precursor polyprotein from which virion core proteins, reverse transcriptase (RT) and integrase (IN) enzymes are derived. The env gene product is a precursor protein from which 'envelop' proteins are derived. These viral proteins localize at the plasma membrane of the infected cell, where crescent shaped structures that develop into virions budded off from the cell may be visualized under election microscope.

4. **Cell transcription and Tumour formation :** The acutely transforming viruses like Rouse sarcoma virus carries 'V one' genes (srcgene) which are responsible for early onset of neoplastic transformation. Src gene encodes on transformation specific phosphoprotein in the infected cell with protein kinase activity. Phenotypic change associated with high levels of this phosphoprotein is responsible for the 'transformed' state (Hanafusa, H. 1989).

Slowly transforming viruses, such as 'Lympohid Leucosis' viruses do not posses a V-one gene but these viruses transform cells indirectly by activation of a cellular C-one gene. ALV provirus gets integrated with the host C-myc clones, which is then expressed under the influence of the viral LTR promoter sequence. The enhanced expression of the C-mye gene by this 'Promotor insertion' is believed to initiate the lymphomagenic process. (Goodenow, M.M. *et al.*, 1990).

"Defectiveness "of some Avian Retro-viruses

A number of avian retroviruses have been shown to have 'defective genomes'. They arise due to either experimental mutagenesis or sometimes spontaneously in nature.

Some acutely transforming RSV strains have lost their 'V-onc' gene, loosing their ability to transform rapidly. They are called as 'transformation defective (td)' mutants. These mutants can produce tumours slowly like 'LL' viruses occurring naturally. Some acutely transforming viruses show defective replication due to the lack of env genes, which are called as replication defective (rd) mutants.

'BH-RSV' strain of Rouse Sarcoma is a classical example of an 'rd' mutant and is used in diagnostic test for Avian Leucosis viruses. This test is called 'Non-producer (NP) cell activation test' it works as follows:

On single infection of chicken embryo fibroblasts (CEF) the defective virus genome of 'BH-RSV' functions to bring about replication of viral RNA transformation of infected cells and production of gs antigen, but only non-infectious progeny particles are produced, which are unable to enter new host cell because they are 'replication defective'. Now if 'non-replication defective' ALV (LL virus) is added to this BH-RSV infected cell culture system, LL virus being 'non-defective' will act as 'Helper virus' for defective BH-RSV and 'Productive' infections BH-RSV will be produced which can be detected in supernatant fluid by assays in susceptible CEF cultures which forms the basis of 'NP' test. In this 'NP' test, BH-RSV viruses of A,B,C,D and J sub-groups are used separately for identification of unknown LL isolate using the above principal.

Strain Nomenclature

Strains of Avian Leukosis/sarcoma group are named according to pre-dominant neoplasm they produce with an affix to indicate their origin with an individual e.g. 'Rouse sarcoma virus (RSV)' or location eg: Regional poultry research laboratory isolate 12 of LLV (RPL 12 – LLV). Substrains of RSV are designated according to individual who studied them, e.g.: the high titred strain of Bryan (BH-RSV), sub-groups (eg: A) may be designated also (PR-RSV-A). General terms avian leukosis virus (ALV) and avian sarcoma virus (ASV) are widely used to designate members of the group.

Helper viruses isolated from stocks of other viruses e.g.: RAVS have been designated numerically (e.g.: RAV-1), where a helper virus is used for replication of a defective virus, this is also indicated e.g.: BH-RSV grown with RAV-1 as helper is designated as BH-RSV (RAV-1). Strain of ALV that acts as resistance inducing factors was designated as 'RIFS'.

Pathogenesis and Eipzootology

Chickens are the natural hosts for all Avian Retroviruses and are not isolated from any other avian species except pheasents, partridges and quails. However, experimental transmission can be made in unusual hosts by passaging in young animals by induction of immunological tolerance prior to inoculation. Thus, Rouse sarcoma has a widest host range.

Immunity

The exogenous ALVS infect most of the chicks in natural field conditions and they develop virus Neutralizing antibodies at high titres and persist throughout the life of birds. These antibodies are passed to progeny chicks via yolk and provide passive immunity to infection for 3 to 4 weeks of age of chick. This delays the ALV infection and reduces incidence of tumour, viremia and shedding of ALV. These VN antibodies, thus limit neoplasia. ALV infected birds also have cytotoxic lymphocytes directed against viral envelop antigens.

Vertical transmission occurs in only few chicks in a flock but the infected progeny chicks becomes a major source of infection to other pen mates or shed mates horizontally. The virus is not thermo-stable outside the live host and hence, indirect contact infection is not important source of infection.

Four classes of infection related serological status are prevalent in any given flock as ALV is quite ubiquitous in the poultry populations. These classes are: 1) No viremia, No antibody (V-A-), 2) No viremia with antibody (V-A+), 3) With viremia with Antibody (V+A+), 4) With viremia, No Antibody (V+A-). Only birds with infection free flocks, such as SPF flocks, category (V-A-) is prevalent as well as in case of genetically ALV resistant birds this category is found.

Most of the commercial flocks show (V-A+) birds in majority while only minority birds (10%) are generally (V+A-). Most V+A- hens transmit ALV to a varying but relatively high proportion of their progeny. A small proportion of V-A+, hence transmit the virus congenitally and do so more intermittently. The cocks act only as virus carriers and source of contact or venereal infection to other birds (hens). Hens shed ALV into egg albumen and with presence of virus in the vagina of hens (albumin secreting glands in oviduct shed virus in egg albumin while egg production).

Usually minority of ALV infected birds develop LL while others remain carriers and shedders of the virus. Viremic tollerent (V+A-) birds are more likely to die of LL than those with antibody (V-A+).

Pathogenesis

The LL is a malignancy of the bursa dependent lymphoid system, which is evident, when bursa removed surgically prevents L.L. in nature also, it is observed that when bursa is atrophied due to IBD infection, incidences of clinical LL are absent or greatly reduced.

Changes in isolated bursa follicles can be observed as early as 2nd week of age of LL infected birds and by 7th week, abnormal follicles are present in bursa of most infected chickens while abnormal follicles in bursa expand and displace adjacent normal follicles until, by 16-24 weeks of age at the earliest, a gross tumour of bursa is visible and metastasis of the bursal tumour through lymphatic system and blood bring about generalization of the toumor in visceral organs.

Immuno-fluorescence studies provide one more evidence that cells of LL tumours, transplantable tumors and lymphoid cell lines cultured in vitro have B-cell markers and IgM on their surface (Payne *et al.*, 1975) and (Neuman and Witter, 1979).

Serotype-2 MDV (example–SB-1 MD vaccine strain) was found to enhance the development of LL in certain feather sexed lines of chickens following exposure to ALV after hatch (Bacon L.D. and Witter, R.L. *et al.*, 1989).

About the Disease

Lymphoid Leukosis: Congenitally infected embryos after hatch or horizontally infected stocks between 1 to 14 days of age show clinical signs of Lymphoid Leukosis only after 14th to 30th weeks of age and occurrence of natural cases of LL below 14 weeks of age are very rare and incidence of LL is highest at about period of sexual maturity.

Affected birds may show paleness shriveling or cyanosis of comb (occasional) lack of appetite, emaciation and body weakness occurs frequently. Enlargement of liver is palpable.

Grossly visible tumors almost invariably involve liver spleen and Bursa of Fabricious. Involvement of other organs like kidney, lungs, gonads, heart, bone marrow and mesentery is variable.

Tumour growth can be nodular, miliary or diffuse or a combination of all these 3 types. Tumors can be spherical or flattened. Liver may show numerous small nodules uniformly distributed throughout the parenchyma. In diffuse form, the organ is uniformly enlarged, with slightly grayish colour and usually friable.

Histopathology

H.E. stained sections of liver may show that all tumours are of focal and multicentric origin. Diffuse tumors show coalescing foci pattern. As tumour cells proliferate, they displace and compress the cells of organs rather than infiltration between them.

Tumour consist of aggregates of large lymphoid cells of almost uniform size (monomorphic) with poorly defined cytoplasmic membrane and have basophilic cytoplasm and a vesicular nucleus in which there is margination and clumping of the cromosomes and one or more conspicuous acidophilic nucleoli. Cytoplasm of most tumors have large amount of RNA which stains red with methyl green pyronin indicating that the cells are immature and rapidly dividing. The most pre-dominant cells are lymphoblasts. Lymphoid Leukosis is the most pre-dominant form of ALC found in the field.

Erytholastosis

This tumour forming disease has long incubation period, when the virus strain lacks viral oncogen and when it has to depend on cellular oncogen for its expression. There is a general anaemia and petechial haemorrhages in various organs like muscles, subcutis and viscera. Thrombosis, infarction and rupture of liver or spleen may be observed along with oedema of lungs, hydro pericardium and sero-fibrinous clots can be seen on surface of liver. The main lesions are diffuse enlargement of liver and spleen or kidneys. Haemangiomas can be either involving all the layers of blood vascular system or only endothelial predominance with cavernous loose tissue containing erythropoetic cells with primitive anaeplastic cells or haemocyto blastic stages of cells.

Nephroma and Nephro blastoma

Leukosis virus induced kidney tumors include Nephroblastic cellular morphology or adenomatous or carcinomatous growths. These tumors can occur in age groups of birds between 18 days to 7 weeks of age. Nephro blastomas are pinkish grey nodules embedded in kidney parenchyma or yellowish grey lobules that replace most of kidney tissue. They can be pednuculated or may be connected to kidney tissue by a thin fibrous vascular stalk or may be cystic in nature. They show tubular structures with invaginated epithelium or malformed glomerular structures. Papillary cyst adeno-carcinomas are also frequently observed.

Hepatocarcinomas

These are primary tumours of liver tissue caused by MC-29 strain of Leukosis virus. They show solid structure less masses of large altered liver cells with irregular contours, vesicular nuclei and large dense nucleoli. They may show almost normal to markedly disarrayed liver cell masses, adenomatous or tubular, mosaic and giant cell arrays, haemorrhagic carcinoma complexes and hepato bilbiary cell process. Metastasis to organs like lung, kidney and spleen can be seen.

Osteopetrosis

This tumour may have an incubation period between a month to 3 months and is caused by RP12-L-29 strain. Long bones of limbs are most commonly affected. Birds with advanced disease have characteristics 'book like' shanks. Affected chickens are usually stunted and they walk with stilted gait or limp.

Gross lesions include thickened periostium and sponginess of long bones, which gives the bone a fusiform appearance. In long standing cases, the periosteum is not as thick as it was earlier and when it is removed, the porous irregular surface of the very hard osteopetrotic bone is revealed. Osteopetrosis and LL frequently occur together in the same bird. There is premature atrophy of bursa and thymus and splenic atrophy can also occur.

Connective tissue tumours

These include fibroma, fibro sarcoma, myosarcoma, osteoma, oasteo-sarcoma and condrosarcoma. These tumours occur sporadically.

Transmission

Exogenous ALVS can be transmitted in two ways, namely vertically from hen to progeny through egg and horizontally from bird to bird by direct or indirect contact.

Studies on Rouse Sarcoma reveal that birds with tumors also have 'tumour Associated Cell Surface Antigens' (TASAS) which serve to retard tumour growth or regression of tumors. TASAS may be viral structural antigens and they may be affected by anti-viral responses or they may be 'neo-antigens' on tumor cells. They may be virus directed and virus specific or they may be host antigens. The 'TASA' may be called as tumour specific transplantation antigens (TSTA) when they induce tumour immunity *in vivo* or as transformation specific cell surface antigens (TSSA) when demonstrated in *in vivo* tests only (Bauer H.R. *et al.*, 1976, Weinberg M.A. *et al.*, 1976, 1985). But in fact, very little is known about immunity in LL.

Genetic Resistance

Genetic resistance to tumour development has been studied mainly with the Rouse sarcoma, regression of which is determined by a dominant gene R-RS-1 that lies within the major histo-compatibility complex (MHC locus) of the chicken and located I the B-L region. Work of Heinzelmann *et al.* (1981) suggests that progressor birds may have on MHC antigen that cross reacts with Rouse Sarcoma virus induced tumour antigen resulting in immune tolerance.

Genetic resistance to LL tumor development, such as in RPL line 6, is conferred by bursal cells, and not by other cellular elements of immune system, such as thymic or thymus derived cells or non-lymphocytes. It appears as though the intrinsic inability of the bursal target cells to become infected or transformed is the major factor in resistance.

Diagnosis

Virus Isolation and Identification of Causative Agent

Virus can be isolated from most soft organs and tumours present on the same from affected bird. Plasma and serum are also the best materials for virus isolation. Oral washings, feces and albumen of newly laid eggs or the 10 days old embryos of such eggs laid by hens transmitting virus vertically are also very good sources for virus isolation.

Inoculation of susceptible chicks or inoculation of embryonated eggs by CAM route can be used for virus isolation, the later procedure is good for fast growing RSV, as it produces pocks lesions on CAM.

However, cell culture inoculation (chicken embryo fibroblast (CEF) inoculation is also used for virus isolation.

For identification of virus thus isolated some diagnostic tests, such as complement fixation (CF), Elisa and possibly non producer (NP) test or fluorescent antibody test (FAT) can be applied.

The resistance inducing factor (RIF) test can be performed only on viruses that are non-rapidly cytopathogenic (e.g. ALVS), other tests are specific for certain virus strains. Rapid transformation of Fibroblasts cultures (CEF cultures) is produced only by certain sarcoma viruses (see Fadly, 1989 Laboratory manual for isolation and identification of Avian Pathogens–American Association of Avian Pathologists for details). The principals involved in some important diagnostic tests for Avian Retroviruses are shown below:

Resistance – Inducing Factor (RIF) test

ALVS do not induce visible cytopathic effect (CPE) in CEF cultures but they (CEF cultures) become resistant to super infection by a sarcoma virus of the same sub-group. Only viruses of the same sub group become resistant with one another in this way. This property of interference is used in RIF test for assay of ALVS and for identification of isolated ALVS sub-group.

In RIF test, known susceptible chicken embryo fibroblast cultures (CEF cultures) are inoculated with unknown ALVS isolated in 4 separate sets and these cultures are sub-passages separately 3 to 4 times at the interval of 3 to 4 days and cells sample of each set is tested for susceptibility to RSV of different sub-group or alternatively, supernatant fluid of each set of infected CEF may be transferred to new cell culture every 4th day. In this case cells may be challenged without sub-culture 4-6 days post inoculation. Presence of ALV in a cell culture is indicated by a 10 fold or greater reduction in number of foci on similarly challenged control cells. Several different challenge viruses, one for each sub-group must be used to detect ALVS belonging to different sub-groups each requires a separate cell culture plate for testing.

Test for viral group specific internal antigens (COFAL test)

Detection of major antigen present in the core of leucosis/sarcoma viruses, known as group specific (gs) antigen in culture of CEF that have been used for unknown ALV isolation from field case, is carried out by complement fixation test (COFAL test) designed specifically for this purpose.

Infected CEF Cells from cultures cultivated for 14 days are harvested and are adjusted to a standard concentration, frozen thawed and then used as antigen in the test, along with similar preparation of non-infected CEF culture cultivated and processed similarly is used as 'control' preparation (use of CEF cells from source of chickens devoid of endogenous ALV is necessary to avoid confusion in this test). Complement fixing antiserum against 'gs' antigen can be obtained from hamsters bearing sarcomas induced by RSV (Schmidt - Ruppin strain is usually used for this purpose). Complement fixation test is carried out as per standard protocol used for CF test (details not given here for want of space).

NP cell activation test

This test is also used for detection of ALV group A,B,C, D and J, using envelop defective strains of RSV (BH-RSV) to produce transformed cells that are non-producers of infections RSV of sub-groups A to D. Super infection of a culture of NP cells by a Leukosis helper virus results in production of infectious RSV which is detectable in supernatant fluid by assay in susceptible CEF cultures, which forms the basis of N P cell activation test (See paragraphs of Defectiveness of certain retrovirus strains described previous in this chapter for additional details).

'ELISA' test

Highly sensitive ELISA test for gs antigens have been developed. Egg albumin or cloacal swab material can be used directly or after inoculation of these materials on CEF culture and incubating for 7 to 9 days, the infected cells can be harvested, frozen and thawed and cell lysates can be used for ELISA test for detection of gs antigen. In this case, Rabbit anti P 27 antibody can be used to coat the ELISA plates as antibody against common ALV antigen (gs antigen). This test is used for detection of ALV positive carriers in control programme for ALV on Breeder farms of hatcheries.

Differential Diagnosis of ALC from Marek's Disease

Avian Leukosis/sarcoma group of Diseases and Marck's Disease are both the tumour forming diseases of poultry. The tumours produced by strains other that LL from Leukosis/sarcoma group can be identified and differentiated easily from Marek's Disease tumor by histo-pathological differences in the microscopic characteristics of the tumor morphology. However, LL tumours and Marek's tumours have similar gross appearance and hence, need differential diagnosis. The following criteria can be used to differentiate them from each other:

1. Marek's Disease (MD) tumour are generally detectable grossly as early as five to six weeks of age but are generally found in birds from 10-12 weeks of age upto 14 weeks of age. Ordinarily LL tumors do not appear before 14 weeks of age and most of mortality occurs between 24 to 40 weeks of age. However, now-a-days, late Marek's Disease mortality especially in case of VVMD in observed between 18 to 24 weeks.
2. Bursal tumours are invariably present either big or small in lymphoid leucosis (LL) but may be totally absent and bursa is atrophic in MD. However, if tumour is present in bursa in case of MD, there is infiltration of lymphocytes in interfollicular space while bursal tumour in case of LL shows presence of large Lymphocytes with vesicular large nuclei in intra-follicular space.
3. Pleomorphic lymphoid infiltration in nerves, cuffing around small arterioles in white matter of cerebellum and lymphoid cell infiltration of feather follicles in skin are characteristics of MD and are not seen with LL.
4. LL tumours microscopically show typical monomorphic, homogeneous population of lymphoblasts in contrast with MD tumors which show pleuomorphic small to large size Lymphoid cells and plasma cells and Marek's Disease cells.
5. LL tumor cells are highly 'pyroninophilic' while medium and small lymphocytes that predominate in MD tumours are not pyronino-philic and do not get stained with pyronin, when stained with Methyl green pyronin.
6. LL tumors are almost entirely composed of B lymphocytes, characterized by IgM surface markers, where as 60-90% MD tumour cells are T lymphocytes which lack IgM markers and only 3-25% cells in MD tumour are 'B' lymphocytes which show

IgM markers on their cell surface. In addition 0.5 to 35% MD cells have tumours associated cell surface antigen (MATSA) which is absent from LL tumour cells.

Prevention and Control of ALV

Immunization

Use of antiviral vaccines to increase host resistance is very attractive but Burmester (1968) demonstrated that attempts to inactivate the LL virus preparations to induce antibodies against LL failed due to the destruction of ability of antibody production cuncurrantly during the inactivation process. Attempts to produce attenuated strains of virus that do not induce disease have also failed (Okazaki, W. *et al.*, 1982). Some attempts to increase resistance of the host to Rouse Sarcoma Virus (RSV) by immunization with viral or cellular antigen were successful (Bennet D.D. *et al.*, 1987 and Payne, L.N. 1981). Similar approach to study of immunization to LL is warranted. Recent attempts for expression of sub-group A envelop glycoproteins of recombinant ALV have given some hope for potential vaccine production (Mc Bride *et al.*, 1985).

Congenitally infected chicks are immunologically tolerant, however, and thus, cannot be immunized even if suitable vaccines are available and these chicks are unfortunately the major source of virus transmission and they mostly develop clinical LL. This is the main reason for failure of all attempts for development of successful vaccine development against this malady.

Testing and elimination of positive virus carriers for prevention and eradication of this disease

Policy of testing and elimination of positive LL reactors for eradication of this disease was followed only in case of small LL free flocks used for getting SPF eggs for vaccine production upto 1977 due to the expensive, long and complicated methods being used for the same until that time. Since 1977, eradication from commercial flocks has become feasible, using the techniques of Spencer *et al.* The following is the outline only for such eradication principal and technique.

Eradication of ALV infection depends on breaking the vertical transmission of virus from dam to progeny. It is necessary to hatch rear and maintain in isolation a group of chickens free from congenital infection. The procedure for eradication of ALV involves:

1. Selection of fertile eggs from hens negative in the egg albumin or vaginal swab test.
2. Hatching of chicks in isolation in small groups (25-50) in wire-floored cages and avoidance of manual vent sexing and vaccination with a common needle to prevent mechanical spread of any residual infection.
3. Testing of chicks thus reared for ALV by biological assay or PCR on blood, discarding reactors and contact chicks and
4. Rearing ALV free group in Isolation.

In practice selection of hens with a low shedding rate is a simpler requirement to fulfill than the subsequent chick testing and isolation rearing needed for achieving complete eradication. Hence, many hatcheries of commercial breeders are concentrating on reduction of infection rate than complete eradication.

Chicks are more susceptible for contact infection immediately after hatching. Although congenitally infected hatchmates are likely to be main source of such infection, these are several procedures for reduction and elimination of infection remaining from previous populations. Incubators, hatchers, brooding houses and all equipments should be thoroughly cleaned and disinfected between each use. Chick boxes should not be reused and each farm should have only one age group of chickens on the farm.

Avian Leukosis Complex – Indian Scenario

During late fifties, sporadic instances of Avian leucosis (Lymphoid Leucosis) complex, especially 'big liver' disease form was known to the pathologists at Bombay Veterinary College. However, when the author (Dr. S.V. Pandit) worked at Poultry Training Centre, Kolhapur (1962-63), he observed daily significant mortality due to 'Big liver' disease at Govt. Poultry Farm, Kolhapur. The disease prevalence was more pre-dominant in Rhode Island Red (RIR) breed than in case of white leg horn birds and incidence was more in RIR females than in RIR males. The Author got the disease confirmed as ALC on histopathological evidence from Bombay Veterinary College (confirmed by Late Dr. B.L. Purohit then Professor of Pathology at BVC). It seems that this disease was probably brought to India through import of Rhode Island Red and white leg horn birds from USA through 'Technical Co-operation mission USA' at Govt. Poultry farms in India.

Later on during late sixties, lymphoid leucosis with involvement of liver, spleen and kidneys was observed in Arbor Acres layer birds as well as in Rani shever layers in sporadic form. Few sporadic cases of osteopetrotic form of the disease was also observed on Govt. farms in white leg horn birds in those days.

During late seventies, Venkateshwara Hatchery group started 100% testing of their pure line layer breeders which brought down the incidence of Lymphoid leucosis in their commercial layer birds. This helped in improvement of their layer birds egg production performance significantly. However, incidence of LL in various breeding farm in sporadic form in broiler breeders of various commercial Hatchery groups continued to occur which still persists as the breeders carry out only random elisa monitoring in broiler breeder birds.

During early and late nineties, SB1, (Serotype-2) cell Associated MD vaccine was introduced in India for control of suspected VVMD Problems in breeder and commercial birds. Since then there was slight rise of LL problems in broiler birds. It is thought that probably this rise is due to enhancement of exogenous or endogenous ALV expression by serotype-2 MDV originated from the vaccine. Taking into consideration of this possibility, some hatcheries stopped use of cell Associated SB1, MD vaccine in their broiler breeder stocks and their corresponding broiler breeder pure lines.

It was also observed that during early years of the beginning of 21st century (2001 to 2007), sporadic incidences of the LL visceral form (Big liver disease) still continues to be a problem especially in broilers, occasionally bringing about increased incidences and mortality due to stress conditions and immune suppression caused by CAA and Reo Viruses.

Suggested Reading

Biggs, P.M. (1964). The Avian Leucosis Complex. World's Poultry Science Journal, 20(2): 8-91.

Biggs, P.M. and Payne L.N. (1964). Relationship of Marek's disease (neural lymphomatosis) to lymphoid leukosis. Natl.Cancer Inst. Monogr.

17: 83-98. De Boer, G..F., Maas, H.J.L., Van Voten, J. and Groenendal, J.E. (1981). Horizontal transmission of lymphoid leukosis virus. Influence of age, maternal antibodies and degree of contact exposure. A vian Pathology, 10: 343-358.

Burmester, B.R. (1947) Studies on the transmission of avian visceral lymphomatosis. Incidence and Propagation of lymphomatosis with cellular and cell free preparation, Cancer Research. 7: 786-797.

Burmester, B.R., Walter, W.G., Gross, M.A., Fontes, A.K. (1959). Journal of the National Cancer Institute, 23: 277-91.

Chubb, L.G. and Gordon, R.F. (1957). The avian leucosis complex—a review. Vet.

Ellermann, V., and. Bang, O. (1908). Experimentelle Leukamie bei Huhnern. Zentralbl. Bakteriol. Parasitenkd. Infections kr. Hyg. Abt. Orig. 46: 595–609 Reviews and Annotations 3: 97-120.

Furth, J. (1933). Lymphomatosis,myelomatosis and endothelona of chickens caused by a filterable agent. Transmission experiments. J. Expt. Med. 58: 253-275.

Payne L.N., Gillespie A.M., Howes, K. (1992). Myeloid leukaemogenicity and transmission of the HPRS-103 strain of avian leukosis virus. Leukemia. 6: 1167-1176.

Roloff, F. (1868). Mag. ges. Thierheilk. 34:190. (Original not available for examination; referred to by Chubb, L.G. and R.F. Gordon, 1957. Vet. Reviews and Annotations 3: 97-120.

❑❑❑

Chapter 8

Inclusion Body Hepatitis/ Hydropericardium Syndrome

(Leechi Heart Disease): Prevention and Control – Indian Scenario

Preamble

Incidence of inclusion body hepatitis (IBH) without the involvement of heart was reported by Panisup, *et.al.*(1982) as a result of re-activation of otherwise dormant adenovirus infection after severe immune suppression by classical IBD virus infection. This was followed by recording of IBH incidences in U.P. (Srivastava, 1990), Kharole, *et al.* (1991) in Haryana and Khera, *et al.* (1994) in Punjab. Harmeet Singh, *et al.* (1994) studied effects of mycotoxicosis in feed on enhancing the pathological condition caused by IBH virus of Punjab. Balachandran (1993) recorded incidence of IBH in layer flocks in Tamil Nadu with low mortality and involvement of only liver. This was the only incidence in layer birds while all the above mentioned incidences were present in broilers only.

It is interesting to know that all the incidences of IBH infections reported from India mentioned above occurring before 1994 involved only liver, kidney lesions and heart lesions were not recorded. Moreover, the mortality percentage was also low (0.8 to 3.0% only).

During August, 1987, Peculiar disease condition with involvement of heart, liver and kidney was reported from Angara Goth, Karachi, Pakistan by Jaffery (1988) and Hasan (1981) which was named 'Angara Disease'. This disease was characterized by typical hydro-pericardium and hepatitis with basophilic intranuclear inclusion bodies in hepatocytes and resulting into heavy broiler mortality ranging from 60 to 70%. This sort of disease syndrome was not reported previously from any part of the world before subsequently Abdul Aziz *et al.* (1991) reported occurence of such disease with IBH/ Hydropericardium syndrome from Iraq. This syndrome could be reproduced in broilers by inoculation of liver homogenate from Affected birds (Khwaja, *et al.*, 1989), Muneer, *et al.*, 1989 and Afzal, *et al.*, 1991).

After detection of an adenovirus in the liver homogenate Khawaji *et al.*, 1988, Cheema, *et al.*, 1989), some workers (Hasan, 1989) suggested that the disease was inclusion body Hepatitis, caused by Tipton strain of Adneno virus (Type IV). However, different serotypes of adenovirus have been isolated from IBH/HPS affected birds in Pakistan (Saaghy, 1989). Cowen (1992) suggested that IBH/HPS has multiple etiology, including IBD virus, Avian Adenovirus and probably chicken Anemia agent.

During the year 1993, peculiar disease similar to 'Angara Disease' was observed in Jammu & Kashmir and Punjab area adjoining the Pakistan Border. VHL scientists including one of the authors (SVP) visited the affected areas of Jalandhar, Pathankot, Amritsar and Ludhiana District of Punjab in August, 1994 and investigated the disease syndrome. Srinivas Gowda (1994) reported this disease condition from Punjab after investigation in August, 1994. Local farmers described the disease as 'Leechi heart Disease' due to the peculiar appearance of heart similar to de-shelled 'Leechi' fruit.

Etiology and epidemiology

Detailed investigations and experiments with laboratory reproduction of the disease conditions revealed that the disease syndrome is caused by multi-factorial etiology. Aflatoxin containing feed (0.01% toxin), facilitated easy reproduction of the disease in experimental SPF chicks (3 weeks old), after injecting 10% suspension of liver, bursa, spleen, kidneys and hydro-pericardial fluid, from affected birds. However, disease of mild nature and with low mortality could also be produced in SPF chicks which were not treated with afflatoxin indicating that the original agent(s) in the infective material was fairly virulent. The Agar Gel Precipitation Test (AGPT) on original and laboratory reproduced affected tissues revealed presence of IBH and IBD viruses.

It was concluded from experiments conducted that IBH virus which seems to be more virulent then usual dormant Adeno-viruses is a primary causative agent for this syndrome. The viral virulence was augmented after immune suppression caused by IBD virus exposure and/or feed toxicity due to afflatoxin or some other myco-toxins or clostredial and other bacterial toxins.

After initial occurrence of IBH/HPS syndrome in North (1994), the disease was reported from Madhya Pradesh, Odisha and Maharashtra in 1995-96 (study group on Poultry disease: IBD/IBH/ Avian Influenza appointed by Technology Mission on Dairy Development March, 1996-Report). Breeder farms are found to be free from this disease so far, probably due to adequate bio-security measures and good management practices undertaken by them. It is the personal observation of the author that the IBH virus isolates from initial out breaks from Amritsar and North India (1994) were requiring association of immune suppressive agents take afflatoxin or IBD or artificial immune suppression caused by corticosteroid injection along with the field isolate for reproduction of the disease syndrome in laboratory conditions in SPF chickens. However, it was significant to know that the attempts of laboratory reproduction of the disease syndrome with field isolates of IBH/HPS out breaks later on during 1995-96, from Pune and Palladum (Tamil Nadu) out breaks were successful without prior immune suppression i.e. with use of field isolate alone.

After review of the history of recording of IBH incidences since 1982 upto the date in India and above mentioned experiences of the 'Disease reproduction' experiments in laboratory, the Author (S.V. Pandit) likes to believe that "IBH i.e. Adenovirus type IV virus which was having a symbiotic relationship with Broiler birds before 1980, might have started becoming slowly more virulent by 1982 (when Mohanti, *et al.* reported 0.5 to 3% mortality due to this virus) probably due to mild immuno suppressive environment created by classical IBD virus in those days". This IBH virus gained more and more virulence during 1992-93 episode of VVIBD in India and it was able to precipitate 'Leechi Heart' disease in north by 1994, wherein additional involvement of heart in addition to liver started occurring with 60 to 80% mortality. However, reproduction of the disease in laboratory was requiring use of artificial immune suppression as described above. However, the evolution of IBH virus 'to become independent' fully virulent pathogen without the help of immune suppression (natural or artificial) was evident in 1994-95, when its outbreaks occurred in Broiler populations in Pune (Maharashtra) and Palladam (Tamil Nadu). The author (S.V. Pandit) presented this concept in the conference of pathdogists, virologists and immune biologists held at IVRI, Mukteshwar October, 1995.

Symptoms

The disease starts generally between 15 to 18 days of age in broiler chicks and continues for a variable period from 10 to 20 days. Even though no specific symptoms are noted, chicks may exibit ruffled feathers, dropping of wings, severe anaemia or in terms, finally resulting into death. The mortality varies from 20 to 80% and occasionally even upto 90%. It has further been reported that the birds remain active until just before death.

Gross lesions

Accumulation of fluid in the pericardium has been found to be the most prominent macroscopic lesions by most workers (Anjum, *et al.,* 1989, Cheema *et al.,* 1989). Hydro-pericardium is observed in 90% of the dead birds in which the pericardial sac had a balloon like appearance having upto 20 ml of the clear straw coloured fluid. Apart from the hydro-pericardium, other changes include swollen, friable, congested and dark to yellow coloured 'mottled' livers with large areas of focal necrosis and patechial haemorrhages. Pale yellow, soften and friable kidneys and edematous lungs have also been observed. Spleen shows mottling with enlargement or atrophy. The bursa shows hypertrophy, containing slight mucous but atrophy of bursa is also reported. Thymus shows haemorrhages in few cases. The breast and thigh muscles show streaks of haemorrhages similar to IBD lesion while only congestion of the muscles was observed in some cases. Bone marrow is pink but yellowish bone marrow with adepose deposition was also not uncommon.

However, Hydro-pericardium with straw coloured fluid gives typical appearance of 'Deshelled Leechi' fruit gave the local name of 'Leedhy Heart Disease' to the syndrome.

Histopathological changes

Zenker's degeneration of heart muscles with eosinophilic and vacuolated cytoplasm with interstitial oedema is prominent. The Haemorrhages and endothelial proliferation of blood vessels in heart muscles are also prominent. The liver parenchyma shows severe degenerative changes with basophilic intra-nuclear inclusions. However, 'acidophilic' inclusions are some times reported. There is infiltration of inflammatory cells, especially of mono-nuclear type. The kidney sections revealed nephrosis i.e. there are severe degenerative and necrotic changes in epithelial lining of kidney tubules with hyline casts in their lumen and there are haemorrhages observed in interstitial tissue of kidney parenchyma. Degenerative and necrotic changes in germinal centers of spleen are also observed. Moderate depletion of lymphocytes in thymus lobules with haemorrhages is also evident. Bursal plicae show oedematous changes in inter-follicular tissue and moderate depletion of lymphocytes in the follicles. Cystic changes in follicles are also observed in late cases. Occasionally haemorrhages are also noted in the follicles.

Disease Incidence

Mortality from 20 to 70% and many times upto 80% is observed in affected broiler flocks. Even though incidence of the disease is mainly in broiler flocks, occasionally layer flocks were also found affected in north zone. Disease occurs in age group of 3 to 6 weeks in general but earliest affection was observed in 15 to 18 days age also. Mortality lingers on for 3 to 6 weeks.

Preventive and control measures

The disease having multi-factorial etiology, it is necessary to prevent immune suppressive predisposing factors, such as:

i) Avoid feed containing afflatoxin in significant level. Use of soya cake in feed instead of groundnut cake as latter may be containing higher levels of Afflatoxin.

ii) Avoid use of contaminated 'offal meals', blood meals or improperly sterilized meat meals in feed which may be containing clostredial or staphylococcal toxins.

iii) Checking of immuno-suppressive viral disease agents, such as IBD, Reo and Marek's Disease viruses. IBD virus subclinical incidence which can occur during 1st week of age of broiler chicks bring about precipitation of IBH infection by even at 18th day at the earliest use of IBD (Luckert type strain) vaccination in 1 to 3 day of age may help avoiding immune suppression and hence, precipitation of IBH infection in early age.

iv) Use of ½ dose of Marek's Disease (MD) vaccine in one day old broiler chicks helps reduction in incidence of IBH as MD vaccination protects them from immune suppressive effect of early Marek's Disease field infection (Generally broiler chicks are not vaccinated against MD on economic ground by commercial broiler farmers).

v) Practicing Bio-security measures and proper heat stress management including supply of clean water throughout the day. Use of vitamin C, A, D_3 and E in proper proportion will also be useful in immune modulation and prevention of Leachy Heart Disease.

Vaccines

During the 1st phase of IBH/HP syndrome incidences in North India, no commercial vaccines were available for prevention of the disease (1994 to 1996). However, the private practitioners started use of liver triturate, inactivated with formaldehyde (Source of liver was the dead birds from affected farms with liver and heart lesions) as 'autogenous' vaccine. This practice even though gave limited success for prevention of Leechi heart disease empirically, it produced more harm to the poultry industry, as there were possibilities of precipitation of other unknown and known diseases on those vaccinated farms due to inadequate and uncertain inactivation of used tissue which were many times affected with other diseases like ND, IB, IBD and salmonellosis, *E. coli*, etc. This practice which was originated in Pakistan proved practically harmful to poultry industry in Pakistan due to flaring up of ND, IB and IBD infections in that country.

However, systematic propaganda against practicing Autogenous vaccination by ignorant farmers and quacks was launched by various hatcheries in India which proved useful in prevention of catastrophe in India. Moreover, Autogenous Vaccine produced by following scientific norms for preparation of such vaccine until the 'licensed' vaccine was made available by private companies also paid fruitful in prevention of this malady.

The author (S.V. Pandit) was working with Ventri Biological Division of Venkateshwara hatcheries and he made successful attempts for isolation of IBH adenovirus in SPF chickens and production of Master seed from such liver tissue isolate which was shown to contain only Adeno virus type IV, without any other contaminating extraneous pathogen (in the year 1996).

Use of such purified master seed of IBH/HPS virus was made for Production of Vaccine virus brew in commercial oil adjuvanted vaccine production. Ventri Bio could obtain license for production of commercial IBH/HPS formalin indivated, oil adjuvatned vaccine after submission of data on 5 field trials designed by this author. This was the incidence of development of such vaccine against this malady for the 1st time in India and this was the 2nd licensed vaccine in the world against IBH/HPS, (1996), 1st vaccine being manufactured in Mexico (1996) few months before our vaccine was presented.

The licensed vaccine on IBH/HPS when used in the field, it proved almost 100% successful and by the end of the year 2000, the incidence of IBH/HPS almost disappeared from Indian scenario.

However, off late some incidences of reemergence of the IBH/HPS or only IBH have been occasionally reported. But it requires detailed investigations to know whether these incidences are due to real vaccine failure or due to some other inadequacies or due to emergence of mutant antigenic variants or there are different serotypes involved in such instances.

Suggested Reading

1. Afzal, M. and Ahmad, L. (1990). The veterinary record 126: 59-60.
2. Afzal, M. *et al.* (1990). Etiology and control of hydro-pericardium syndrome in broilers in Pakistan. Proceedings of 3rd international Veterinary congress, Islamabad, Pakistan 218-228.
3. Afzal, M. *et al.* (1991). Studies on etiology of hydro-pericardium syndrome (Angara disease) in broilers. The veterinary record 128: 591-593.
4. Ahmad, I. *et al.* (1990). Efficacy of formalized liver organ vaccine against Angara disease in broiles. Veterinary Arkhiv 60: 131-138.
5. Khan, A.A. *et al.* (2005). Hydro-pericardium syndrome in Pakistan: a review, world poultry science journal Vol. 61 (December, 2005).
6. Panisup, A.S. Mohanti, G.C. & Verma, K.C. (1982). Indian Journal of Vet. Pathology 6: 24-28.
7. Deepak, J.N., Katariya, J.M. K. Dhama, R. Somvanshi and Verma, K.C. 'Pathogenecity of Fowl Adeno-virus serotype-4' isolated from case of Hydro-pericardium Syndrome. Indian J. Comp. Microbiol. Immunol, Infect Dis. Vol. 25:1 (Jan-June 2004): 7-13.

8. Survshe, B.D., Pandit, S.V., Ghalsasi, G.R. and S. Mallikarjun 'Inclusion Body Hepatitis/Hydro-pericardium syndrome (Leechy Heart Disease)' in India. An Overview Proceedings: World Poultry Congress, New Delhi, India 2-5 Sept., 1996 : Vol. II, pp. 375-379.

9. Report of study group on 'Poultry disease: infectious Bursal disease', Inclusion body Hepatitis and Avian Influenza, Appointed by Technology mission on Dairy Development, March, 1996, pp. 14-18.

❑❑❑

Chapter 9

Egg Drop Syndrome-1976 (EDS 76)

Egg drop syndrome (EDS 76) is characterized by healthy looking layer birds producing drop in egg production with thin shelled or shell-less eggs and is caused by an haemagglutinating adenovirus infection.

The egg drop is characterized by failure of birds to attain a peak of production or 'peaking' birds showing a fluctuating drop in egg production.

EDS 76 was first described by Van ECK, *et al.*, 1976 in Holland. Mac Ferran, *et al.* isolated an haemagglutinating adenovirus in Ireland in 1977 from egg drop syndrome in layer poultry birds. Yamaguchi, *et al.* (1981) isolated adenovirus from egg drop problems in Japan while firth *et al.* recorded the isolation of this virus from Australia also in 1981. It is Mohanti, *et al.* (1984) who were the first to record the egg drop syndrome with shell-less eggs in India during 1984.

About the virus

Egg drop syndrome 76 virus is an adenovirus, classified on the basis of its morphology, replication and chemical composition. The avian adenovirus group antigen is not detected by AGPT or Immuno-fluorescence and there is a shared group (common) antigen between other avian adenovirus infections and EDS 76. EDS 76 is not related to 11 fowl and 2 turkey prototype adenoviruses, using SN or HAI tests.

Using preparations made from cesium chloride density gradient, typical triangular faced morphology, having six capsomeres on the edge and single 25 nanometer fibro projecting from each vertex was demonstrated.

About the Disease and Its Spread

It appears that the virus is transmitted vertically and horizontal transmission of the disease does not occur from flock to flock in the field. The virus remains latent until birds approach the peak of production of eggs quite often. The classical disease depends upon the re-activation of latent virus around peak production, thus establishing a strong association between the age of the flock and the onset of clinical signs.

As the growth of EDS 76 virus in chicken embryo fibroblasts and in chicken eggs is limited and there is no growth in turkey egg embryo fibroblasts and in mammalian cells while there is maximum growth of the virus in duck embryos and duck embryo fibroblasts and as there was absence of any antibodies to EDS-76 before 1974 in chickens, it is postulated that this was probably a virus of duck origin before 1974. The virus was probably introduced in chickens through a contaminated vaccine. Could it be Marek's vaccine HVT-FC-126 produced on Duck embryo fibroblast culture.

As the disease is transmitted vertically, there is an apparent association of the breed with this disease. Spread occurs quickly probably due to relatively quick breakdown of number of carriers at once at a time. The endemic EDS spreads often by contaminated egg trays, transport workers and materials in case of classical outbreaks.

The sporadic outbreaks of EDS-76 occur as a result of chicken becoming infected through direct or indirect contact with infected wild or domestic water fowl. The disease and the virus has no public health significance. The disease is characterized by sudden drop of production of eggs which comes to normal within 15 days to one month period. The egg shells become thin and fragile while number of shell less eggs also increases to higher side. The egg drop of infectious bronchitis virus, after sudden drop, does never come back to normally. While EDS egg drop comes back to normalcy after course of the disease ends which is the typical differentiating character between EDS and IB.

Gross and Microscopic Lesions

Only inactive ovary and atrophied oviduct are the gross lesions seen in the EDS. Microscopic lesions are not characteristic.

Diagnosis

Proper evaluation of the egg production charts and sero-monitoring of antibodies using HAI test (showing rise in HAI antibodies in recovery stage sera samples as against acute stage sera samples) is of diagnostic value for establishing the adeno virus EDS as a cause of Egg drop condition.

Prevention of EDS by Vaccination

In endemic areas, the disease can be prevented by use, of an inactivated oil adjuvanted vaccine given at 14th to 16th week along with proper bio-security and disinfection measures.

EDS 76: Indian Scenario

After establishing the presence of EDS-76 in India by B.S. Mohanty, *et al.* (1984), Egg Drop Syndrome as a result of haemagglutinating EDS-76 adeno-virus was recorded by scientists of Venkateshwara Hatcheries group in north, in Punjab and Haryana in late nineteenth century years in Hyderabad and vizag–Ananparthy poultry belts in Andhra Pradesh by them.

V.H. group undertook a project on EDS-76 vaccine production after serological survey using HAI test for sero-monitoring of this adeno-virus infection during 1987-1990 sponsored by 'NABARD'. Formalized inactivated oil adjuvanted EDS-76 vaccine was developed using duck embryo fibroblast cultures for propagation of EDS-76 adeno-virus. The virus was also grown on chick embryo fibroblast cultures of SPF egg origin for producing vaccine against EDS-76 on commercial level. However, the occurrence of EDS-76 infection in the field was not sufficient enough to embark upon actual production of this vaccine on commercial scale.

❑❑❑

Chapter 10

Chicken Infections Anaemia

Chicken Infectious Anaemia is a newly emerging highly immune suppressive disease of young growing chickens characterized by aplastic anaemia and generalized atrophy of haemopoetic lymphoid tissue with resultant subcutaneous/intramuscular haemorrhages on breast or thigh muscles of the chicken. Yousa, *et al.* (1979) recorded this disease in Japan for the 1st time, followed by its incidences in February (1980) and other European countries. Chettle, *et al.* (1989) described the occurrence of this disease has spread all over the world in chickens. Yousa, *et al.* (1980) demonstrated the effect of maternal antibodies in day old chicks on the susceptibility to the Chicken Anaemia Agent (CAA). It is shown that CAA is vertically transmissible from the infected parents (breeder hens) to the progeny chicks. The maternal antibodies (MAB) from such affected breeder hens can also be transferred simultaneously to the progeny chicks. The Chicken Anaemia Agent (CAA) gets positively affected due to the presence of MABs simultaneously present in day old chickens and gets suppressed. After waning of the MAB titers in 3 to 4 weeks, the chickens become susceptible to CAA virus again and CAA infection flares up either due to the re-activation of suppressed CAA virus or fresh CAA virus re-infection. McNulty, *et al.* (1988) in a longitudinal survey of 2 broiler breeder flocks, demonstrated that maternal anti-CAA antibody persisted until about 3 weeks of age and both flocks get sero converted to CAA at 8 to 9 weeks of age.

Symptoms of the disease

The affected chicks exhibit anorexia, lethargy, droopiness and pale coloured body with severe anemia. The disease in its clinical form can be seen in 1st week (it can be seen from day one onwards) in the flock, when it has originated from the vertical transmission sometimes, followed by 2nd cycle in 4-6 weeks age in the same flock due to the waning of MAB. The disease virus can spread by vertical transmission in day old chicks from the breeder hens as well as it can spread horizontally in the pen-mets. Mortality varies from 5 to 15 per cent. Following primary infection in breeder flocks, disease chicks are produced for 3 to 6 weeks suggesting the time of multiplication of virus in breeders and development of antibodies in serum which appears to prevent further egg transmission (McNulty, 1994). The effects of this disease in broilers include depletion of the lymphoid system resulting into depression of the cell mediated immune response, exposing the birds to secondary economic performance of the broilers.

Subclinical CAA infection can persist longer time and it can bring about severe immune suppression resulting into secondary bacterial infections (Calneck, *et al.* 1991), such as precipitation of clostridium perfringens or clostridium choevei and staphylo-coccus infections of wings or skin with lesions of severe cellulitis and wing rot or gangrenous dermatitis with sero sanguineous exudates accumulation. This condition is also described as 'Blue wing disease.' Simultaneous IBD infection can also contribute to the severeness of CAA immune suppression. The unattended flocks with Anaemia-dermatitis syndrome can suffer mortality of 10 to 60%.

CAA infections at early stages of life of chickens depress protective vaccinal immunity of HVT vaccine given at day one stage and can bring about precipitation of Marek's Disease outbreak, simulating the one due to Natural very virulent MD (VVMD) outbreak caused by VVMDV which occurs in spite of HVT vaccination. This observation is mimicked experimentally by reproduction of severe MDV infection after simultaneous inoculation of CAA and VMD isolate together in HVT vaccinated one day old chicks (Otaki, *et al.* 1989). They also demonstrated that pathogenecity of CAA was enhanced by infectious bursal disease virus (IBDV) at one day, 14 days, 21 days and 28 days age and Atrophy of the thymus and aplacia of bone marrow were more severe in chicks with dual inoculation that the one inoculated with CAA alone.

Lesions of CAA

The CAA is known to cause thymic atrophy resulting in immune suppression and increased susceptibility to other infections causing a complex problem. Along with thymus, Bursa of fabricious and spleen also get atrophied and the bone marrow is also affected with atrophic haemopoetic lymphoid tissue and gets replaced with fatty tissue resulting into 'yellowing' of bone narrow. Sometimes, bone narrow becomes 'watery' with blackened discolouration. The thymic lobes show paleness with petechiel hemorrhages and drastic atrophy of lobes. Histo-pathological examination (microscopic) revealed 'rarification' of the medullary portion of thymic lymphoid follicles with fibrous tissue replacement followed by adipose tissue infiltration in medulla of bone narrow. The haemorrhages are also observed in thymic follicles. The Bursa of fabricious shows changes similar to those observed in case of IBD infection. The germinal centers of the spleen show paleness and lymphoid atrophy.

The peripheral Red blood cell counts are drastically reduced and the haematocrit values are drastically affected with severe anaemic changes. Many times the bird becomes icteric with paleness of comb (or icteric comb) and pale shanks. RBC sedimentation volume is drastically reduced (Haematocrit value < 27%).

About the virus

Classical review of CAA by McNulty (1991) describes CAA as a DNA viral entity belonging to the family circoviridae, with 20-30 nm un-enveloped (naked) icosahedral capsid composed of one polypeptide and containing a single stranded circular DNA approximately 2.3 KD molecular weight. All CAV isolates isolated so far belong to one pathotype and one serotype only.

Incidence of Chicken Infectious Anaemia (CIA): Indian Scenario

1st reported incidence of Chicken Infectious Anaemia (CIA) was recorded by Tamil Nadu Veterinary and Animal Science University (TANUVAS) in 1993, giving evidence of histo-pathological findings on 45 specimens and isolation of virus from 6 specimens.

During the investigations of incidences of VVIBD outbreaks during its 1st phase in Tamil Nadu (1993), the Author (SVP) came across the lesions of Thymic atrophy and thymic haemorrhages in large number of IBD incidences, during the post mortems of IBD affected carcasses. This is in addition to all typical IBD lesions. The Author attributed these thymic lesions to VVIBD. However, now author feels that these thymic lesions might have been due to combined CAA and IBD super-infections and that is why even 99% mortalities occurred during those days. The contemporary findings of CAA during 1993 by 'TANUVAS' scientists support this author's view, though not attempts of the confirmation of this view.

The author recorded clinical and histo-pathological evidence of occurrence of CAA outbreaks in Bombay, Pune poultry belt since September, 1997. However, clinical and histo-pathological findings of CAA infection were confirmed by serological evidence by the author in Ahmednagar in July, 1998 and in Pune poultry belt in August, 1998. Incidences of 'Runting and Stunting Syndrome' with thymic Atrophy in layer grower birds with serological evidence of CAA were confirmed in Ajmer Poultry belt in Sept., 1998 followed by similar instances in Barasat and Bongaon (West Bengal), 24 pargana (South) district near Bangladesh border in 1999 (March-April). In the same year similar incidences were recorded in Jalandhar, Berwala, Gurgaon and Jind in Punjab and Haryana and in Hyderabad in the months of May to August. It was revealed during all above investigations that the mortality due to CIAV varied from 10% to 20%. Even though clinical manifestation of the disease is limited, sub-clinical infection produces severe immune suppression due to affection (atrophy) of thumus, bursa and spleen leading to reduction in response to ND, IB, IBD, vaccinations to subsequent precipitation of mycoplasma, choryza and fowl pox and ND, IB infections on very large scale in those poultry belts mentioned above. This CCRD or RDC (Respiratory Disease complex) problem does not yield to any antibiotics.

The Marek's Disease incidences in North and some poultry belts in Hyderabad and Bangalore (including Mysore) as well as in Pune (involving not only the commercial poultry but also the breeder farms) were significantly increased with the characteristics simulating 'VVMD+' like severity in both commercial and breeder poultry flocks, during recent out breaks in the year 2005-06. These affected flocks also showed presence of CIAV clinical picture (further confirmed Histo-pathologically and serologically) prior to MD incidences (Age 60to80 days for CIAV and Age 12 to14 weeks for Marek's manifestation). The investigations indicate that CIAV produced severe immune suppression which resulted into failure of immunity of even the cell Associated HVT + Cell Associated SBI vaccinations in Breeders chicks as well as commercial chicks administered at day one stage at Hatchery level and booster vaccinations carried out from 4 days to 18 days post hatch at farm level.

The increased incidences of CIAV has resulted in severe economic losses to poultry farmers in terms of mortality, reduced weigh gains in broilers, egg production losses in layers and increased cost of medicines.

The incidence of CIAV mentioned above was observed in all the breeders in India. This may be due to the possibility of spread of CIAV infection through CIAV contaminated vaccines produced on 'Non-SPF' ordinary eggs produced indigenously, or some sub-standard imported 'CIAV' contaminated vaccines can also be the culprits. Incidences of accidental contamination of CAA infection in SPF flocks and subsequent contamination of live vaccine(s) produced on such contaminated eggs from SPF flock are already recorded in Germany and Japan.

Control of CIAV through Vaccination

Even though Bio-security is the best way for prevention of infectious diseases, CIA infection is not easy to control through Bio-security/Disinfection programme only as CAA is very sturdy and thermo-stable virus and it does not get killed by formaldehyde or lime powder very easily.

However, the maternal immunity can prevent the chicks from clinical disease and immune-suppression, when they are present in the chicks. Hence, the progeny of the breeder flock, vaccinated with live vaccine at proper age, is immune to CAA infection upto 3-4 weeks. It is, therefore, necessary to immunize the parent stocks against CIAV for proper control of the infection in commercial flocks upto 4 weeks of age.

E. Vielitz, V.V. Bulow and C. Conrad of Lohmann Tierzncht GMBH, Cuxhaven, West Germany reported production of live CAA vaccine produced from live field isolate (CUX-1) passaged in CAA susceptible SPF egg embryos. The vaccine virus titre on MSB1 cell culture was 4 to 5 TCID 50/dose which is equivalent to 100 chick infective doses (50%), i.e. 100 CID 50/dose.

The experimental trial with this vaccine concluded as follows:

1. It is known that grower birds of 12 to 16 weeks of age are resistant to CAV infection. Hence, this is the ideal age for vaccination against CAV with safety as in the case of AEV infection.
2. Breeder birds are vaccinated between 12 to 16 weeks of age with above live CAA vaccine.
3. Breeders develop solid immunity against CAA after 3 weeks post vaccination.

4. The progeny chicks of the immunized breeders were found to be resistant to challenge CAA infection.

The infected flocks are vaccinated in Germany with CUX-1 strain vaccine of Lohamann GMBH as described above to obtain commercial progeny resistant to CAA during the early age. This avoids the immune suppressive effect of field infection of CIAV during early chick life. It is expected that ND, IB, IBD and MD immunizations are carried out during the 1st 4 weeks of chick's life and hence, passive immunity against CAA during this period is useful in avoiding any bad effects on development of immunity against MD, ND, IB and IBD infections. Moreover, as chicks are in growing phase, they start becoming resistant to CAA infection naturally.

Vaccine Production in Indian Context

Presently, no official CAA vaccine is available in India and the importation of any live CAA vaccine is also banned. Production of experimental inactivated CAA vaccine for 'in house field trials' is reported by the commercial vaccine manufacturers are in process of getting the live or inactivated vaccine licensed. Till then, the control of the presently deep rooted Immuno suppressive scenario in Indian poultry is a big question mark. (Indian Situation, 2005-16).

Suggetsted Reading

Mcnulty, M.S., Connor, T.J., Mcnilly, F., Kirkpatick, K.S. and Mcferran, J.B. (1988). A serologicalsurvey of domestic poultry in the United Kingdom for antibody to chicken anaemia agent. Avian Pathology, 17: 315-324.

Yuasa, N., Taniguchi, T., Yoshida, I. (1979). Isolation and some characteristics of an agent inducing anemia in chicks. Avian Diseases; 23: 366-385.

Yuasa, N., Noguchi, T., Furuta, K. and Yoshida, I. (1980). Maternal antibody and its effect on the susceptibility of chicks to chicken anaemia agent. Dis., 46: 945-955.

❑❑❑

Chapter 11

Avian Reo Virus Infection: Newly Emerging Pathological Disease

Entity with Multiple Clinical Expressions

Avian Reo Viruses are prevalent worldwide, being found in most commercially reared poultry populations and probably in many other avian species as well.

Avian reoviruses are incriminated as the etiological source for diverse clinical manifestations including viral arthritis, femoral head necrosis, tenosynovitis, maladsorption syndrome, 'Runting and Stunting' syndrome, proventriculitis, gizzard erosions, poor feathering (helicopter syndrome), liver damage, respiratory disease. However, more than one etiological factors were found involved in these complex syndromes in various geographical areas. Individual reovirus isolates may differ in disease producing ability with same isolates being quite pathogenic while others are relatively innocuous. Frequently, the virus can be isolated from the respiratory and intestinal tracts of otherwise normal birds.

Reoviruses were first identified as avian pathogens in by Olson (1957), however, this viral agent was identified as Reovirus by Petek, *et al.* (1967). Involvement of viral agent in tenosynovitis in chickens was demonstrated by Rossi, *et al.* (1969). Fahay and Crauley (1954) isolated virus from chronic respiratory disease of chickens. Above mentioned identification of this Fahay-crawley viral agent as Reo virus was pointed out by Petek, *et al.* (1967). Deshmukh and Pomeroy (1969) carried out isolation and serological characterization of Avian Reoviruses from intestinal tract of chicks with cloacal pasting. They showed that this isolate when inoculated in susceptible chicks produced teno-synovitis. Avian reovirus could be isolates from teno-synovitis and arthritis lesions as well as from 'ruptured tendons' by Bottino (1975) from Italy, Glass, *et al.* (1973) from USA, Johnson and van der Heide (1972) from Maine (USA), Jones, *et al.* (1975) from U.K. Thus, workers from U.S.A., Europe, South America and several other countries have reported incidence of Teno-synovitis due to Reo virus infections in poultry.

It has been found that in the field, if broiler breeder flocks experienced clinical signs of teno-synovitis well before egg production started (usually around 7 weeks of age), their broiler progeny had very little, if any, clinical problems or plant condemnations due to teno-synovitis by AGP testing of breeder flocks for the presence of reovirus antibodies, it was observed that correlation appeared to exist between a negative AGP status for reovirus of the parent flocks and the development of clinical teno-synovitis in the broiler progeny. The presence of maternal antibody against reovirus seemingly afforded protection of progeny chicks against teno-synovitis.

A disease syndrome of broiler chickens characterized by stunted growth (Runting and stunting syndrome, RSS), increased feed conversion (Maladsorption syndrome) and poor feathering (Helicopter chick disease) was initially reported in Netherlands by kowenhoven, *et. al.* (1993). The syndrome has been described as Femoral Head Necrosis and 'Infections proventriculitis'. The clinical signs and pathological lesions are variable. The affected flocks show a growth depression to the extent of 25% to their otherwise healthy penmets (McNulty, 1993). Rosenberger (1983) demonstrated isolation and characterization of Reosvirus from young commercially reared Delmarva broiler chickens affected with stunted growth, arthritis, abnormal feathering, osteroporosis and lack of pigmentation of shanks and increased mortality in U.S.A.

Symptoms Exhibited in Various Reo viral Infections

A. Teno-sinovitis and viral arthritis

1. Swollen knee joints (bilateral swelling) are observed in broiler parents as well as commercial broiler birds at 6-8 weeks of age. The tendons also show accumulation of synovial fluid in their sheaths.
2. The affected joints and their tendons make the joints immovable.
3. Birds cannot reach upto their feed and hence start becoming under weight.

B. Femoral Head Necrosis

This condition is seen in both broiler and layer flocks and the affected grower layer birds are unable to walk. The post mortem examination reveal damaged femoral head cartilage with raw bleeding surface.

C. Runting and stunting syndrome

This condition is seen in commercial broiler grower chickens. The first appearance of beginning of Runting is observed as early as 5 to 7 days of age. 1 to 40% of the broiler chickens in the infected flock show the marked reduction in body weight while the rest of the individuals in the flock exhibit normal size and body weight. Mortality in affected flock varies from 0 to 15 per cent. Age 1 to 28 days post hatch is the most vulnerable age for this syndrome. Poor feathering with abnormality in the structure of feathers bring about 'helicopter appearance' of the affected chicks. This happens only in case of 'infected' chicks while the normal sized healthy birds show the normal pattern of the feathers. There is abnormal dis-colouration of the shanks but it is not a constant finding. Wet litter is observed in number of broiler flocks affected with Runting and stunting. Mucoid diarrhoea is seen in 5-10% affected birds with undigested particles in faeces.

Post mortem findings

Abnormalities in size of proventriculus which is enlarged and showing thinning of the proventricular walls and swollen proventricular papillae with increased secretion of muco purulent discharge flowing out of proventricular gland's papillae is observed in some outbreaks of Runting and stunting but not in all the outbreaks. Haemorrhagic papillae are also seen in some cases probably in outbreaks complicated with CAA or NDV infections.

Intestines are swollen, distended with poorly digested feed; histo-pathological findings include pancreatic vacuolations, cystic dilatation of crypts of Liberkhun and Necrosis of Crypt epithelial cells (Kowenhoven, *et al.,* 1983). Histological examination of jejunal tissue shows a reduction in the number and density of intestinal villi responsible for absorption. The ultra structural studies of enterocytes revealed Entero like viral particles.

The Bursa of fabricious shows marked atrophy. Thymus may be normal but our observation in Runting and stunting syndrome in Ajmer revealed atrophy of thymus, probably due to complication of the Reo virus infection with superimposed CAA infection (Rise in antibody titers against both Reo and CAA infection by ELISA testing were recorded in this case).

Abnormalities of Rib cartilage are reported from Holland, Germany and Israel (I.D. Jaspers and K. Rudds of Intervet Dupher Holland, March, 1985). Femour and shank bones show rubbery elasticity with naked articular surfaces without cartilage cover completely or partially (observations in Bashirhat and 24 Pargana South district, 2001).

About the virus

Avian Reo virus belongs to the family *Reoviridae* and is a DNA virus which is a non-enveloped virus with icosahedral symmetry with a double capsid. The information from cross protection studies and challenge studies indicate that reoviruses examined thus, far are similar antigenically to S 1133 (viral arthritis) isolate. This could be important in the development of vaccines since a Single Serotype may induce protection against a wide range of reovirus pathotypes mentioned in this chapter previously.

The article entitled 'Immunity of just hatched Broiler chicks' from Maternal antibodies in various Concentrations against Reo virus infection (viral arthritis) by Kouwenhoven, *et al.* (1988) from Netherlands mentions that inactivated vaccine (Nobivac, Intervet, Boxmeer the Netherlands) comprises the American strain 1733 and 2408 isolated by Rosenberger from broilers with maladsorption syndrome. These isolates share common antigens with the Connecticut isolate 51133 which is a chicken embryo adapted Tenosynovitis producing Reo virus strain (Van der Heide, *et al.*, 1975).

Vaccines and Vaccinations

Two types of vaccines are available for protection against Reo-virus infections abroad:

1. Inactivated oil adjuvanted Reovirus vaccine containing 2 American strains 1733 and 2408 which were isolated by Rosenberger *et al.* from 'Maladsorption syndrome' which share

common antigens with 'Connecticut isolate' of viral arthrithis 51133. This vaccine can be used at prelay age (18-22 weeks) of the broiler breeding flock and it can be repeated at Mid-lay (40-45 weeks of age). This can be sufficient to take care of the maternal antibody requirement of progeny commercial broiler chicks produced by the breeder flock throughout the laying period from 22-24 week onwards upto the disposal of the breeder flock.

2. Chick embryo adapted (attenuated) live Connecticut 51133 strain (highly egg embryo passaged virus (73rd passage level) reovirus vaccine, freeze dried applied subcutaneously is capable of inducing immune response even in the presence of maternal immunity (MAB) which declines substantially by 15 days of age of chicks. Chicks with MAB vaccinated at 10 or 25 days of age provide good immune response by 3rd to 4th week of age.

Reovirus Infections: Indian Scenario

1st recorded incidence of Reovirus associated with viral infectious Arthritis in poultry in India is by Kataria, *et al.* (1985) followed by work on reovirus by Kataria., Mohanti, *et al.* (1986). Mallikarjun and Kataria (2003) showed that Avian Reovirus isolated from proventriculitis is non-enveloped virus with icosahedral symmetry and double capsid.

The author (S.V. Pandit) recorded incidences of clinical 'helicopter syndrome' in broiler commercial chicks of 3 to 5 weeks of age during his routine field visits to Namakkal (Tamil Nadu) for investigation of incidences of VVIBD outbreaks in 1993-94. Possibility of involvement of immune suppression by VVIBD subclinical infections might be responsible for precipitation of this probable Reovirus manifestation.

Bhardwaj, *et al.* (2003) recently demonstrated that CAA agent and Reo virus when experimentally co-infected, can produce severe teno-synovitis which coincides with our field observations as far as another manifestation of Reovirus infection, namely 'Runting and stunting syndrome' in layer commercial birds, which we observed in Ajmer poultry belt during the year 1998 (September). Atrophy of thymus with high CAA antibody titres along with reovirus titres were noted during this 'Runting and stunting' episode which was found in that poultry belt on 'wide spread' scale and with 50 to 60% runting and stunting, which is quite severe and high.

Viral arthritis in commercial broilers and broiler breeders at 6 to 9 weeks of age due to reovirus infection is reported in early 21st century (Year 2000 to 2006) period. Runting and stunting with maladsorption syndrome and helicopter syndrome is also recorded in various poultry regions in the country recently (years 1992-93, 1999-2000 and 2003 to 2005), wherein serological evidence of Reovirus infection was recorded by the author (S.V. Pandit) with other scientists of V.H. group (Ventri bio and PDRC, Loni). The experimental vaccines (inactivated) produced from the local isolates used in trials on 'in house' flocks' revealed successful control of the local incidences. Presently, farmers are using 'imported' inactivated vaccines which are not authorized by the Govt. machinery. The applications for licencing the indigenous inactivated Reo Vaccine production are still on processing line and need urgent action for their approvals.

Suggested Reading

Bhardwaj, N., Kataria, J.M., Dhama, K., Arthur, S.S. and Sentilkumar, N. (2003). Ind. J. Comp. Microbiol., Immunol. And Infec. Dis., 24: 2.

Deshmukh, D.R. and Pomeroy, B.S. (1969). Avian reoviruses. I. Isolation and serological characterization. Avian disease 13: 239-243.

Fahey, J.F. and Crauley, J.F. (1954). Studies on chronic respiratory disease of chicken II Isolation of virus, Can. J. Comp. Med 18: 13-21.

Perk, M.B. *et al.* (1967). The Crauley agent An Avian Reovirus Arcoh ges. Virusforsch 21: 414-424.

Glass, S.E., Naqi, S.A., Hall, C.F. and Kerr, K.M. (1973). Isolation and characterization of a virus associated with arthritis of chickens. Avian Diseases, 17: 415-424

Johnson, D.C. and van der Heide, L. (1971). Incidence of tenosynovitis in Maine broilers. Avian Diseases, 15: 829-834.

Jones, R.C., Jordan, F.T.W. and Lioupis, S. (1975). Characteristics of reovirus isolated from ruptured gastrocnemius tendons of chickens. Veterinary Record, 96: 153-154.

Kataria, J.M., Mukherjee, S.C., Rehbinder, C., Verma, K.C. and Mohanty, G.C. (1985), Electron Microscopic Characterization of a Viral Agent isolated from Arthritis in Chicken.Zentralblatt für Veterinärmedizin Reihe B, 32: 361–367.

Kouwenhoven, B., Vertommen, M. and Goren, E. (1988). Investigations into the role of reovirus in the malabsorption syndrome. Avian Pathology, 17: 879-892.

McNulty, M.S. (1993). Reovirus. In Vims infections in birds (J.B. MeFerran & M.S. McNulty, eds). Elsevier Science Publishers BV, Amsterdam, 181-193.

Olson, N.O. and Weiss, R. (1972). Similarity between arthritis virus and Fahey-Crawley virus. Avian Diseases, 16: 535-540.

Obson, N.O. *et al.* (1957). Infectious synovitis control by medication, effect of strain differences, Avian J. Vet. Res. 28: 735-739.

Petek, M., Feiluga B., Borghi, G. & Baroni, A. (1967). The crawley agent: an avian reovirus. Arch. ges. Virusforsch., 21: 413-424.

Rosenberger, J.K. *et al.* (1983). Role of avian reoviruses in maladsorption syndrome. Proc. 32nd West. Poult. Dis. Conf. 39-40.

Rossi, C., Babini, A., Beccaria, E. and Guarda, F. (1969). Un episodio di tenosinovite virale dei polli. Ricerche virologiche ed istologiche. Atti della Societa Italiana delle Scienze Veterinarie, 13: 1049-1052.

Rosenberger, J.K. (1983). Characterisation of reoviruses associated with a runting syndrome in chickens. International Union of Immunological Societies Proceedings. No. 66. University of Sydney, Australia, 141-152.

Van der Heide L., Kalbac M. & Hall W.C. (1976). Infectious tenosynovitis (viral arthritis): influence of maternal antibodies in the development of tenosynovitis lesions after experimental infection of day-old chicks with tenosynovitis virus. Avian Dis., 20: 641-648.

Jasper Ing, D. Ruddk (March, 1985). Maladsorption, do we speak the same language on both sides of the Atlantic. Document of Int. Vet. Serv. Deptt. of B.V. P.B. 2 1380 A.R. Weesp Holland Salisbury Charles city town.

❑❑❑

Chapter 12

Avian Influenza

Avian influenza is an acute zoonotic and fetal disease of birds with significantly high mortality and morbidity. The disease is caused by virus belonging to family *Orthomyxoviridae* and is characterized by multiple haemorrhagic lesions in upper respiratory and alimentary tract with mucosal inflammation. However, there are no pathognomic lesions or symptoms which can specifically differentiate this disease from other disease of poultry. Avian influenza was first identified in Italy in 1878, in an epidemic of poultry. However, the causative agent was identified as 'Virus' in 1901 by Centanni and Savonuzzi. The disease, Avian influenza was known to the old veterinarians as 'Fowl plague' described in text book of pathology by Geiger and Devis (Editions 1955-60) as 'Fowl plague' which was reported in the Netherlands in 1925-27.

The disease occurred in U.K., in 1956 in ducks, in Scotland (1959) in chickens and ducks. It was reported in USA in Turkeys in Wisconsin in 1965-66 and in Massachusetts, in 1965 and in Canada (Ontario), in 1968. Avian influenza was also prevailing in chickens in Germany, in 1949 and Ukraine in ducks, in 1963, in Czechoslovakia, in 1956, in Australia, in ducks in 1983 and U.S.A. again in 1983-84. At the end of 20th century in late nineties (1997), highly pathogenic 'bird-flue' virus was reported in poultry and ducks with few human cases (18 cases) in Hong Kong, followed by similar incidences of Highly Pathogenic Avian Influenza (HPAI) in China, Thailand, Vietnam (in 2003-2004 and 2006) and Indonesia, China and Japan in 2005. The HPAI virus Pathogenecity was so high that the disease spread rapidly and many European and middle east countries were also affected due to HPAI in poultry though human cases were not reported during 2006 in those countries including France, Denmark, Netherlands, Austria, Albania, Azerbaijan, Bosnia, Herzegovina, Bulgaria, Croatia, Germany, Georgia, Greece, Hungary, Italy, Poland, Romania, Russia, Serbia, Slovakia, Sweden, Switzerland, Ukraine, Iran, Iraque, Africa, Nigeria, Cambodia, Cameroon and India, Pakistan, Afghanistan and Myanmar, etc. (Table 1).

Table 1 : AI viruses involved in epidemics in poultry in the world are tabulated below:

Sr. No.	Year of AI incidence in Poultry/Country involved	Virus strain involved	Pathotype of virus	Whether human cases involved	No. of human effective death
1	1878 / Italy	Virus etiology Proved in 1901	HPAI	No	--
2	1927 / Netherlands	Chicken/H70N7	HPAI	No	--
3	1949 / Germany	Chicken/H10N7	LPAI	Yes	--
4	1956 / England	Duck / H11N6	LPAI	No	--
5	1954 / Egypt	Chicken /	LPAI	No	--
6	1959 / Scotland	Chicken / H5N1	LPAI	No	--
7	1956 / Czechoslovakia	Duck / H4N8	LPAI	No	--
8	1961 / Africa	Tern / H3N3	LPAI	No	--
9	1963 / Ukraine	Duck / H3N3	LPAI	No	--
10	1965 / Massachusetts (USA)	Turkey / H6N2	LPAI	No	--
11	1966 / Wisconsin (USA)	Turkey / H9N2	LPAI	No	--
12	1968 / Ontario (Canada)	Turkey / H8N4	LPAI	No	--
13	1973 / Germany	Duck / H2N3	LPAI	No	--
14	1976 / Alberta (USA)	Duck / H12N5	LPAI	No	--
15	1977 / Maryland (USA)	Gulls / H13N6	LPAI	No	--
16	1976 / Alberta (USA)	Duck / H1N1	LPAI	No	--
17	1982 / Guryev (Europe)	Duck / H14N5	LPAI	No	--
18	1983 / Australia	Duck / H15N8	LPAI	No	--
19	1983-84 / USA	Poultry / H5N2	HPAI	No	--
20	1974 / Memphis USA	Duck / H1N9	LPAI	No	--
21	1963 / Ukraine	Duck / H3N8	LPAI	No	--
22	1972 / Australia	Sea water / H6N5	LPAI	No	--
23	1997 / Hongkong	Chicken / H5N1	HPAI	Yes	18 / 6(33%)
24	1998 / China (main land)	Chicken / H9N2	LPAI	No	--
25	1999 / Hongkong	Quail / H9N2	HPAI	Yes	
26	2003 / Hongkong	Chicken / H5N1	HPAI	Yes	2/1 (50%)
27	1993 / Mexico	Chicken / H5N2	LPAI	No	--
28	1993 / Mexico	Chicken / H5N2	HPAI		
29	1994 / USA	Chicken / H7N2	LPAI	--	--
30	1995 / Pakistan, Nepal, Burma	Chicken / H7N3	HPAI	No	No
31	2002,2003 / USA	Chicken / H2N2	LPAI	Yes	2/0
32	2003 / Netherlands	Chicken / H7N7	HPAI	Yes	89 / 1(1.1)
33	2003 / Pakistan	Chicken / H7N3	HAPI	No	No
34	2004 / Canada	Chicken / H7N3	HPAI / LPAI	Yes	2/0 (0.0%)
35	2003-04/ Thailand, Vietnam, Korea	Chicken / H5N1	HPAI	Yes	52 / 39 (75%)

Sr. No.	Year of AI incidence in Poultry/Country involved	Virus strain involved	Pathotype of virus	Whether human cases involved	No. of human effective death
36	2004 / Hongkong, China, Thailand, Vietnam,	Chicken / H5N1	HPAI	--	--
37	2005 / Indonesia, Laos, Malaysia, Japan, Korea, Zimbabwe	Chicken / H5N2	HPAI	--	--
38	2005 / Magnolia, Kazakhstan, Japan, Russia, Romania, Thailand, Turkey, Ukraine	Chicken / H5N1	HPAI	--	--
39	2006 / Afghanistan, Albania, Azerbaijan, Bosnia, Herzegovina, Bulgaria, Cameroon, China, Croatia, Denmark, Egypt, France, Georgia, Germany, Hongkong, Hungary, India, Indonesia, Iraque, Iran, Israel, Italy, Jordan, Japan, Malaysia, Myanmar, Niger, Nigeria, Korea, Pakistan, Poland, Romania, Russia, Philippines, Serbia, Slovakia, Slovenia, Sweden, Switzerland, Thailand, Turkey, Ukraine, Zimbabwe	Chicken / H5N1	HPAI	--	--

Symptoms

The symptoms are variable from outbreak to outbreak. There can be sudden deaths without any symptoms shown by the birds or there can be severe respiratory distress with muco-purulent nasal discharge, facial oedema, simulating swollen head syndrome, severe coughing, diarrhoea and sometimes characteristic swollen combs with cyanotic patches or haemorrhagic sinus formation in the subcutis of combs. Mortality may vary from 10 to 15% to 90-100% according to the pathotype of the virus (Low pathogenic Avian Influenza (LPAI) Pathotype or Highly Pathogenic Avian Influenza (HPAI) pathotype) sudden 'egg drop' was observed in laying hens affected with A.I.

Lesions

The lesions are characterized by severe subcutaneous and mucosal haemorrhages in various parts of the body with oedema in sub mucosa. The haemorrhagic tracheitis with muco-purulent plugs in trachiea was observed invariably during the postmortems carried out by us during the incidences in India.

Presence of haemorrhages surrounding Proventricular papillae with oedema and hyper secretion of proventricular glands through proventricular papillae was noted in many carcasses but were not as constant symptom as described under 'fowl plague' in old text books as characteristics 'Pathognomic' lesion only pinpoint haemorrhages on proventricular papillae were seen instead many times confusing the diagnosis as 'New castle disease'. Hepatitis showing swollen fragile liver with pinpoint white necrotic foci on liver surface, simulating the liver lesions of fowl cholera was also observed frequently. Haemorrhagic enteritis was often present as prominent postmortem lesion. Flaccid hemorrhagic ova in laying hens was a constant feature.

About the virus

Avian Influenza virus belong to *Orthomyxoviridae* family with eight segments of single stranded RNA molecules contained within the viral envelope in tight association with the Nucleoprotein (NP) and the 3 polymerase proteins (PB_2, PB_1 and PA) which form the ribonucleoprotein (RPN) complex. A.I. virus belong to 'Type A' influenza virus.

The Haemagglutinin (HA) and Neuraminidase (NA) glycoproteins are present on the surface of envelope. The NS, protein is truly non-structural protein and is not packaged in the virion. This NS, protein has a key function of interfering with the cell's anti-viral defense and thus it can be a target for viral attenuation which can be useful in 'anti-flue attenuated vaccine production'. Avian influenza virus has 15 major distinct sub-types based on HA glyco-proteins surface antigens (H1 to H15) and 9 minor distinct subtypes based on NA glyco-proteins surface antigens (N1 to N9) as described previously. All 15 HA and 9 NA subtypes are maintained in the natural host reservoir of wild aquatic birds, primarily ducks, shore birds and gulls.

The virus from migratory birds is shed through their faeces into the nesting places around the water reservoirs on their way of migration and it is caught by the wild ducks in the contaminated water and such infected ducks can carry the virus to the neighbouring village back yard poultry. In countries like Thailand, Vietnam and Cambodia, the farmers take domestic ducks to their rice field to pick up left over of rice crops to clean up the fields. These ducks pick up virus brought by migratory birds and spread in the rice fields where in the sparrows and pigeons pick up this virus and transport the same to commercial poultry farms/backyard poultry birds.

The poultry birds, thus affected shed their virus in the litter. The virus can spread in poultry through contaminated water or even the shedding of virus through the respiratory tract in mucous secretions is possible. The dust in the farms can get contaminated and such contaminated dust can produce aerosols which can spread infection from one poultry farm to another farm nearby.

AI virus is considered avirulent and it is in relatively evolutionary statis in the wild birds. However, when this virus infects a new host species, it can occasionally cause disease and then quickly gets adapted to the new host species, if given the opportunity. HA proteins in particular has been shown to have a rapid rate of evolution in variety of species including humans, swine, chickens and turkeys due to the result of a strong selection pressure for the virus to become better adapted to its new host species as well as due to the host immunologic pressure, e.g. in U.S., live bird markets provide a favorable environment for mutation of AI viruses due to animal movement dynamics of these markets. These typically sale variety of avian species including chickens, turkeys, guinea fowls, quails, ducks, etc. for human consumption and new birds are continuously introduced into the markets. AI virus once entered in such dynamic situation, cycle of infection is maintained. Retrospective genetic analysis of H_7N_2 and H_5N_2 isolates proved this hypothesis during the year 2000 and 2003 out breaks in U.S. Recently quails have been proposed as a potential intermediate host in the spread of AI virus in poultry. Furthermore, a human avian recombinant containing the surface glycoprotein genes of a quail virus and internal genes of a human virus replicated and transmitted readily in quail, raising concern that quail could be a foundation as amplifier of influenza virus re-assortants that have potential to infect humans. However, quails importance in the natural ecology of AI virus transmission is still unclear. Ecological studies have revealed that a vast influenza virus gene pool for A.I. type A virus perpetuates among migratory ducks and their nesting lake water in nature. It is now proved that influenza viruses preferably replicated in the columnar epithelial cells of colon without any disease signs and are excreted in faecal material in high concentration of ducks and deposited in lake water. It is interesting to know that influenza virus isolates from faecal samples of ducks in their nesting areas in Siberia phylogenically belonged to Eurasian linkage and were closely related to those from birds, pigs and horses in Asia. It was noted that these isolates closely correlated to H5N1 influenza virus isolates from chickens and Humans. HA of H5 influenza isolates from ducks in Japan revealed close relationship with H5N1. AI viruses from Hongkong, South China, Thailand and Vietnam and also to H5N1 of ducks nesting in Siberia. It is interesting to know that pigs are theorized to act as 'reaction vessel' of mixing and recombining of Avian influenzas. HA and N genes from chickens and further passage of recombinant genes from pigs to human beings and the rapid spread of H5N1 from chickens to humans in south-east Asia (Thailand, Korea, Japan, China and Hongkong) in 9 years from 1997 to 2006 can be explained with this theory as Duck-Chicken pigs human are typically closely associated. The disease caused by AI virus in poultry can range from asymptomatic infection, local mild infection to systemic replication (infection) which differentiates the causative A.I. virus into LPAI (Low pathotype) to HPAI (high pathotype). This difference depends on the cleavage of haemoglutinin (HA) molecule HA into HA1 and HA2 subunits by host proteases which determine infectivity and spread of the virus. Thus, HA molecule of LPAI can cleave only in certain tissues (limited infectivity) while HA molecule of HPAI has a capacity to cleave in multiple tissues bringing about systemic infectivity. This explains why LPAI can bring only respiratory localized affection while HPAI can cause severe systemic infection in poultry.

AI viruses do not typically replicate efficiently in humans, thus not allowing direct transmission of AI virus from poultry to human being. However, since 1997, several cases of human infections with certain subtypes of AI especially H5N1 (e.g. In Hongkong 1997) and H7N7 (e.g. in Netherlands in 2003) have been recorded.

Originally definition of Avian Influenza (AI) included only highly pathogenic strains (HP) of H5 and H7 serotypes under 'list A' disease according to office international des Epizooties (OIE). However, recently it was observed that most of the H5 and H7 viruses are low pathogenic (LP) strains but some of them can mutate even by single point mutation in HA gene to become highly pathogenic (HP) strain and hence, all the H5 and H7 subtype strains are now considered potentially dangerous and are included under 'List A' disease agents of O.I.E. Thus, chapter 2.7.12 in terrestrial Animal Health Code of O.I.E. define standards for international trade which include definition for poultry notifiable avian influenza (NAI) free establishments. Code defines HPAI as viruses that have an Intra Venous Pathogenecity Index (IVPI) in 6-weeks old chickens greater than 1.2 or which causes at least 75% mortality in 4 to 6 weeks old chickens infected intravenously. It also recommends that H 5 and H 7 viruses which do not comply IVPI greater than 1.2 or cause less than 75% mortality should be sequenced to determine whether multiple basic aminoacids are presents at the cleavage site of HA molecule and if the amino acid motif is similar to that observed for HPNAI isolates, the isolate should be considered as HPAI.

How much is the threat of Human Pandemic caused by Avian Influenza (AI) strain is real?

As mentioned above, Avian strain of influenza from affected chicken can rarely infect human being directly as there are no surface epitopes on A.I. virus which have an ability to attach to the surface epitopes on human cells, as against the fact that HA glycoprotein epitopes of A.I. virus has ability to attach on surface epitopes of chicken respiratory/intestinal tracts columnar epithelial cells specifically. However, it is shown that viral RNA responsible for HA epitopes of H5, H7, HPAI and sometimes, H9 LPAI undergo point mutation at the molecular level and resulted into changes in terminal aminoacid sequences of these epitopes (i.e. known as antigenic drift). Sometimes at unpredictable intervals, viruses with completely different surface antigens or subtypes to which host has little or no immunity are introduced by 'segment re-assortment'. This is known is Antigenic shift. Accumulated antigenic drift due to point mutations may be tolerated in poultry to some extent but not tolerated in humans. Such antigenic drift may make HA epitope of AI virus to get affinity towards human columnar epithelial cell surface for attachment and thus, human cells can become susceptible to A.I. virus with successful occurrence of A.I. infection. However, survival of these antigenic shifts/ drifts requires integrated concentration of duck-poultry-pig-human populations and hence, such chances are very rare. However, it is seen since 1997 after Hongkong incidence that chances, though rare, are still possible to come into reality. However, even though during the period of 9 years from 1997 to 2006, affection of A.I. infection from birds to human (Via. Pigs/quails) totally 204 cases have occurred and 113 persons died. No full proof human cases of infection were recorded upto the date. This phenomenon has occurred in south-east (Asia Pacific) zone only. The Indian experience of early 2006 clearly shows absence of human occurrence in spite of affection of A.I. in poultry.

The chances of A.I. virus infection occurring in human through eating of poultry and their products in countries like India are remote as compared to the same in countries of Asia Pacific region, such as Thailand, Cambodia, China, etc. as their eating habits are different (e.g. they eat even raw poultry/pig meat). It can be noted :

1. A.I. virus can be surely killed by boiling poultry meat at 100^{0}C for more than 30 minutes (cooking), which is far above the WHO safety standards (70^0 C for 15 minutes).
2. HPAI infected hens will invariably die due to the disease and/or stop laying eggs or by shell less eggs which are never marketed. Hence, question of eating infected eggs does not arise and eggs are generally boiled/fried or omleted before eating and no chance of infected eggs becoming available in the market due to above mentioned reasons.
3. A.I. virus is very fragile and gets killed easily by normal disinfectants like formal dehyde, chlorine, gluteraldehyde and many more chemicals and sunlight.

It should be noted that Asia pacific countries have very close connection of live poultry birds markets with duck, quails, pigs and habit of consumption of raw poultry/pig meat is unique in those countries in contrast to the Indian scenario, thus the chances of completion of Ducks - Poultry-quail-pig-human link favourable for antigenic drifts/shifts in HPAI resulting into emergence of mutant HPAI communicable to human being are high.

Symptoms of A.I. Infection in human cases

HPAI symptoms in humans are neither uniform nor predictable and not always over serological surveys have shown that infections with H5N1 in south-east Asia are more extensive than diagnosed by clinical examination (i.e. serological evidences without clinical symptoms were extensive). Only clinical symptoms seen were mild conjunctivitis or transitory malaise and rise in body temperatures. Mortality rate in 52 diagnosed cases in Thailand and Vietnam in recent outbreaks in 2005-06 was higher (75%) while it was lower in 1997, in Hongkong outbreak (35% out of 18 diagnosed cases), suggesting increase in virulence probably due to genetic changes in virus during the spread of infection and rise in poultry population during last 9 years in this region. The scientists express possibility of fatal human pandemic due to newly evolving hybrid strains of A.I. mainly based on these statistical observations. However, even though possibilities of this cannot be ruled out totally, it seems that scientists seem to have over cautioned the fact to much higher scale, if we take into consideration the size of available data on global meager incidences of A.I. which is quite meager as seen above. As a matter of fact, the human incidences of some other zoonotic diseases like Rabies, brucellosis, Anthrax, hydatid disease, tuberculosis are much more higher but have never been spread to Pandemic dimensions.

Incidence of A.I. in India

The neighbouring countries like Pakistan, Nepal and Burma were hit by this malady during 1995, wherein H7N3 subtype was involved. This was repeated in the year 2000. However, H9N2 and H7N3 were reported in Pakistan, in 2003.

During the period of 1995 to 2003, no official report of A.I. was declared by Indian Government. However, Govt. of India attempted to establish facilities for diagnosis and serological surveys for A.I. at High Security Animal Disease Laboratory (HSADL), Bhopal. Facilities of National Institute of Virology, Pune of ICMR were also used for serological survey for 'Type A' Influenza Viruses during this period.

Taskforce for suggesting measures for control of emerging diseases of poultry was also established by Govt. of India (of which the author (SVP) was a member) during this period. They recommended to strengthen the HSADL (central facility) and also to establish specialized laboratory facilities at regional level for the diagnosis and survey facilities for detection of emerging and re-emerging poultry diseases including A.I.

During this period from 1995 to 2003, no official A.I. was detected in India. However, large number of cases of new castle disease with respiratory symptoms including swollen head, sinusitis and haemorrhagic tracheitis were recorded and during the year 2004-2005, number of poultry disease diagnosticians raised a doubt of Avian influenza in north, especially in Barwala, Jind, Panipat, Sonepat Poultry belts and in Hyderabad-Karimnagar–Kurnul poultry belts in south in such respiratory affection of poultry. However, due to the lack of reference Diagnostic laboratories and facilities, disease A.I. remained undiagnosed in India upto the year 2006.

However, during the 4th week of January, 2006 (27th January) the shocking news of occurrence of Avian influenza in Navapur (Dist. Nandurbar) poultry belt was flashed by most of the T.V. channels and it was confirmed on 18th Feb., 2006 as 'H5N1 HPAI' by HSADL, Bhopal and finally endorsed by O.I.E. This was followed by 2nd confirmed report of its occurrence in Jalgaon district (Marul and Savada) on 14th March, 2006 and 28th March, 2006 (Varad: Aldhi, Bhadgaon, Parola, Erandol and Uttarna) in Jalgaon District of Maharashtra and Icchapur–Bwchanpur (in M.P.) and 3rd report on 4th/5th April, 2006 (Pachora and Nandgaon, etc.) and 18th April, 2006 (Janve, Jalgaon and Ichkheda (Maharashtra). Govt. of Maharashtra immediately declared these A.I. incidences as scheduled list A disease as per O.I.E. guidelines from concurrence from Govt. of India and undertook the action of 'Stamping out' of the disease by mass destruction of poultry birds in 10 km radius of the declared areas of the occurrence of the disease followed by deep burial of the same in trenches with disinfectant lime powder. Movement of poultry birds, eggs and poultry products from affected areas was banned, Disinfection and cleaning up of infected sheds was also undertaken. Vaccinations were not allowed to be undertaken. The last case of A.I. was reported on 18th April, 2006 after which no official cases were reported. During the period of poultry, AI outbreaks and even after it, no human cases (clinical or sub clinical /serological) could be detected/diagnosed.

Control of A.I. Epidemics in Poultry

Due to the fear of spread of poultry A.I. infection of human being, the global organizations like WHO and OIE have formulated rigid control measures and regulations for implementation by the Government machineries all over the world in a way that the progress of the A.I. infection in poultry will be halted and this will automatically result into avoidance of coming in contact of affected poultry birds with human being. This can be achieved by 2 possible ways, namely: 1) stamping out policy and 2) vaccination policy.

Stamping out policy

This is the oldest method for halting of the progress of the disease by removing total availability of the susceptible host species and cleaning and disinfection of premises of their infected products / waste materials.

This can be achieved in case of A.I. infection by total destruction (depopulation)/slaughter of poultry birds (Both commercial farm birds/backyard poultry birds of all the age groups including chicks, pullets, grower birds, layer birds as well as broiler birds. This also includes the live birds from infected areas, commercial table eggs as well as eggs meant for incubation and eggs under incubation in the hatcheries in infected areas). The total bio-security measures included disinfection of the farm premises, market bird crates, burning of cages and poultry equipment including feeders, waters and farm sheds, etc.

After complete disinfection of infected premises in the affected areas as described above around the 10 km radius of A.I. declared poultry premises, the entry and exit of live poultry birds and their products is to be banned totally and bio-security/disinfection measures are required to be undertake for the next 6 months to avoid re-occurrence of A.I. incidence in the area.

Theoretically, stamping out policy looks very attractive for total removal of A.I. infection but practically it has got various limitations as follows:

1. Even though infected premises are cleaned off from the infection by destruction of live/slaughtered birds and their products including their discharges, etc., the visits of migratory birds in the areas and contamination of natural water source by them is not easy to avoid.
2. Stamping out policy can be successful only in small countries and isolated islands, where entry of reservoir and carrier birds can be effectively controlled but in bigger countries with availability of various routes of entry/exit for reservoir and carrier birds/animals/infection, failure rates will be high.
3. It is also difficult to control aerosols of the infected virus particles in certain seasons like summer and hence stamping out is ineffective.
4. Stamping out policy needs huge financial compensation provision by Govt. agency the cost of which is prohibitive for developing and under developed countries.

Vaccination policy

The world health organization (WHO) and OIE were recommending implementation of stamping out policy for containment of AI infection in poultry and the scientists were averse to use of vaccine for control of A.I. due to knowledge that A.I. inactivated vaccines can prevent clinical disease and death in poultry but it cannot stop the shedding of A.I. virus from vaccinated birds which become asymptomatic carriers/shedders of virulent AI virus if becomes infected with the field A.I. virus.

Mexico was the first to make long term use of Avian Influenza inactivated vaccine during massive A.I. outbreak due to H5N2 strain of HPAI since 1995. The encoding of sequence of 52 Mexican lineage viruses isolated from vaccinated birds between 1995 to 2002 indicated multiple sublineages of H1 and N5 genes. Serological analysis using HAI test and virus Neutralization test showed major antigenic differences among isolates belonging to different sub-lineages. Vaccine protection studies further confirmed the *in vitro* serological results indicating that commercial vaccine was not able to prevent virus shedding, when chickens were challenged with antigenically different isolates. This indicates that multilineage 'antigenic drift' has occurred in the field which was responsible for the persistence of A.I. virus in the field in spite of long term A.I. virus in the field inspite of long term A.I. vaccination. This may be due to 'antigenic drift' occurring under constant vaccination antibody (immune) pressure. This needs to be taken into consideration while selecting the vaccine strain time to time to avoid shedding of virus from vaccinated birds. Thus, it becomes necessary to continuously monitor the field virus shaded by vaccinated bird population and change and select new vaccine seed strain, whenever 'antigenic drift' is detected. This will enable the scientists to use the vaccination policy successfully without shedding of virus by asymptomatic vaccinated birds. This knowledge has enabled the countries like Netherlands to take a decision of adapting vaccination policy for control of A.I. in poultry after November, 2005 H7N7 and H5N1 (Both HPAI) outbreaks since 2003. Dutch Scientist (Virologists) Albert Osterhans after conducting experimental trial proved that if vaccine strain exactly matching to the field strain is used. (This requires continuous monitoring of progress of field A.I. virus strain in poultry birds). Shedding of field virus by birds can be stopped after 2 weeks post vaccination. Netherland was successful in use of such 'Selective vaccine strain' in inactivated vaccine for control of Avian Influenza since November, 2005 and they could lift the ban and declare the country free from Avian Flue since 1st January, 2006. It can be concluded that the effective prevention of infection and reduction of virus shedding by vaccination is possible. It seems clear that the efficacy of the vaccine depends primarily on the antigenic relatedness of the circulating viruses with the strain used for vaccination.

The model vaccine against A.I. should contain enough quantum of antigenic mass and proper antigenicity of the viral strain and antigenic relatedness of the circulating viruses with the strain used for vaccination.

Thus, it is prudent to prepare a vaccine bank to adequately respond to an outbreak with the following selection criteria of the vaccine seed for emergency vaccine:

1. Select viruses closely matching to the base of phylogenic tree for HA protein sequence which may give more cross reactive immunity.
2. Select viruses that grow well in embryonating chicken eggs in order to obtain increased HA/EID_{50} titres which can provide higher antigenic mass cost effectively.
3. Keep all the potential vaccine seed strains in national A.I. Vaccine Seed Bank sequenced as far as HA antigenic part is concerned so that sequence comparison between newly emerging field strains can be determined/completed in shorter possible time.
4. Conduct HI cross neutralization tests with the strains used for the vaccination and if there is significant difference in HI cross neutralization tests with the strain used for the vaccination and if there is significant difference in HI cross neutralization activity, conduct cross protection studies in chickens directly to assess the efficacy of the vaccine.

Concept of 'DIVA' vaccination policy for differentiation of vaccinated birds from infected birds

Lastly, it is recommended that viruses with unusual NA subtypes which may serve as a marker for differentiation of 'Vaccinated' and 'infected' birds may be selected as 'Vaccine seed' virus. In general N_1, N_2 and N_3 subtypes are the most prevalent in poultry and the virus that does not have these NA subtypes will be desirable. This is the concept of so-called 'DIVA Vaccine' e.g. H5N4 or H7N6 inactivated vaccines if used in countries, where H5N1-N2- N3 or H7N7 HPAI are prevalent in the birds, the vaccinated birds can be easily differentiated from birds circulating virulent field viruses H5N1-N1-

N3 or H7N7 virus as vaccinated birds will have antibodies to H5N4 or H7N6 antigens only while infected unvaccinated birds will have antibodies against H5N1-N2-N3 or H7N7, thus enabling the laboratory to differentiate between vaccinated and unvaccinated but infected birds.

However, 'DIVA Vaccination' policy will be good for such differentiation only where the country has enough number of capable laboratories to undertake DIVA differentiation tests. In our developing country as only Bhopal HSADL lab is having such facility, differential diagnosis in desired short time frame is next to impossible presently. In such situation, use of heterologous N subtype vaccine is not of any significance, any it will be less efficient as far as quantitative 'Protective value' is concerned. In fact use of 'Homologous' M and N subtype containing seed virus, such as H5N1 isolate from the field will have full protective capacity (in present Indian A.I. situation context), as it will be able to stop shedding of field H5N1 virus more efficiently in the opinion of the authors, even though Govt. of India has stockpiled some DIVA vaccine (H5N2 vaccine) for use in recently recorded H5N1 outbreak in India (probably due to non-availability of Homologous H5N1 inactivated/or autogenous vaccine during January, 2006 outbreak.

Dr. Pradhan from HSADL, Bhopal have recently declared that effective H5N1 inactivated vaccine is not developed by HSADL, Bhopal and they may think of giving their strain for vaccine production to the suitable Govt./private sector agency who have high disease security vaccine production facility. Such autogenous inactivated vaccine against HPAI strain (like H5N1) will have to be produced/ handled in high disease security environment only.

The scientists from developing countries are now tending towards the use of vaccination policy for control of A.I. as 'stamping out' policy for eradication of the disease in Thailand, China, Korea and Hongkong has virtually failed. This is obvious due to the fact that those countries with number of available routes of spread of the infection such open air with dusty storms, uncontrollable visits of migratory ducks, wild birds, crows, sparrows, pigeons, pigs, quails, vast backyard poultry population, it is difficult to eradicate the infection inspite of de-population of farm birds and their products.

It is now high time that Government and Private vaccine companies and scientists should come together on common platform and develop long term plan for monitoring the A.I. virus behaviour in nature and react promptly by developing matching vaccine virus seeds time to time for future and produce suitable vaccination bio-security-disinfection plans to fight out A.I. and it's not only for safety of providing population but also for health of humanity because of its predicted pandemicity for humans.

Suggested Reading

Centanni, E., Savonuzzi, E. (1901). La peste aviaria I & II, Communicazione fatta all'accademia delle scienze mediche e naturali de Ferrara.

□□□

Chapter 13

Avian Encephalomyelitis

Avian encephalomyelitis (AE) is an infectious viral disease of young chickens characterized by ataxia and rapid tremors of limbs, head and neck. Hence, the name 'Epidemic tremors'.

Jones, E.E. recorded the 1st outbreak of avian encephalomyelitis (AE) in 2 weeks old commercial Rhode island Red chicks with tremors in 1930, followed by 2 outbreaks in 1st week and 4 weeks old flocks of chicks originating from the same breeder flock in 1932, in 'New England' area of U.S.A. During the next 2 years (1933-34) many more outbreaks were recorded in Connecticut, Massachusetts and main states in USA. The disease was reproduced in susceptible chicks by inoculation of brain material filtrate from field cases in 1934 by Jones, E.E. indicating the viral etiology of the disease. Schaaf prepared the first inactivated AE vaccine for the immunization against AE in 1955. However, calnek *et al* was the first to clarify the epizootology of the disease in 1960 and developed orally administrable live vaccine for the same. Tannock and Shafren (1985) purified AE virus and characterized the virus. Avian encephalomyelitis occurs virtually worldwide (Tannock and Shafren, 1994).

About the virus

AE is classified as an enterovirus belonging to the family *Picornaviridae*. It is an RNA virus with 3 virus specific proteins (VP 1 to 3) with molecular weights 43,000, 35,000 and 33,000 respectively i.e. similar in size to those of polio virus. The virions are 'non-enveloped' with hexagonal profiles and 24-32 nm in size. The virus has five fold symmetry with 32 or 42 capsomeres. It has sedimentation co-efficient of 1485 and is resistant to chloroform, acid trypsin, pepsin and DNASE and is protected against heat by divalent magnesium ions.

All isolates of AEV are serologically similar. There are two distinct pathotypes of the virus, namely:

1. Natural enterotropic field strains which infect chickens readily via the oral route and are shed in faeces. The natural field strains are relatively non-pathogenic except in susceptible chicks infected by vertical transmission or by early horizontal transmission in which case they show neurological symptoms. These symptoms can also be produce by the intracerebral inoculation of susceptible chicks with the natural strains.
2. Embryo-adapted strains constitute the other pathotype, which are highly neurotropic and cause severe neurologic symptoms after intracerebral inoculation or sub-cutaneous inoculation. However, they can't infect even the susceptible chicks via oral route and they can't spread horizontally. These strains are the result of adaptation after multiple passages in antibody free chicken embryos (as a result of probably selection of 'laboratory mutants'. The example is van roikel (VR) embryo adapted (150 passages) strain.

Both the pathotypes can replicate in embryos derived from susceptible flocks. However, the 'natural pathotype' do not show any obvious sign or gross lesion in egg embryo after inoculation by yolk sac or any other route. The commercial AE live vaccine virus strains being 'Natural pathotype' strains do not show any gross lesions in SPF egg embryos after inoculation by yolk sac route and hence, it is not possible to know the titre of AE live vaccine virus by embryo inoculation and opening the eggs for determination of EID_{50} titre. It is necessary to hatch the eggs inoculated for AE live vaccine virus titration and determine the 'Chick Infectivity' titre by detection of hatched chicks observed 10 to 15 days post hatch.

The embryo adapted pathotype strains (like van Roiekal (VR) strain) used in inactivated vaccine production, show typical muscular dystrophy and immobilization of skeletal muscles as gross embryo-lesions especially after 18th day of incubation (after inoculation of six day SPF old egg embryos). This is in contrast with 'no gross lesions seen' in case of Natural pathotype strains used for live AE vaccine production.

Epizootoloy

AE is essentially an enteric infection. Ingestion is the usual portal of entry. Virus is shed in the faeces for a period of several days and it remains infectious for long periods of time, as it is quite resistant to environmental conditions and heat. Young chicks when infected shed the virus for more than 2 weeks in faeces, while chicks above 3 weeks of age excrete the virus for only about 5 days. Infection spreads rapidly from bird to bird and pen to pen or house to house, once introduced, through formites and workers. The disease spread is more likely to be rapid on farms with multiple age groups. Vertical transmission is very important means of virus transmission, based on field evidence and experimental results. Taylor and Schelling reported that 57% of breeder flocks tested in North America had been exposed to the virus by 5 months of age. However, 96% were serologically positive by 13 months.

When susceptible flocks are exposed after sexual maturity, the hens infect a variable proportion of their eggs. Calnek *et al* showed that infected embryos and chicks come from eggs laid during 5 to 13 days after experimental infection of susceptible breeders. The hatchability of eggs from an infected flock is not affected (Jungherr and Minard,1942). However, Taylor, *et al* (1955) observed high embryo mortality during the last 3 days of inculcation. Only chicks from the group with depressed hatchability showed signs of AE. Chicks hatched prior to and after affected hatch appeared normal.

Studies conducted by Calnek, *et al.* (1960) demonstrated that the incubation period in chicks infected by embryo transmission was 1-7 days, whereas chicks infected by contact transmission or oral route had a minimum incubation period of 11 days.

About the Disease

In natural outbreaks, it usually shows its appearance in chicks of 1-2 weeks of age. They show dullness of eyes, followed by progressive ataxia from in co-ordination of the muscles, which is enhanced when by exercising the chicks. Chicks then show inclination to sit on hocks. If disturbed, they lose control over their gait. Finally, they go into lateral recumbancy. Some may still walk on their hocks and shanks. Fine tremors of the head, neck and limbs may be evident, frequency and magnitude of the same may vary. Finally, prostration and death follows. Some individuals with the continued signs may survive and grow to maturity or in some survivors develop blindness due to opacity with bluish discolouration.

The marked age resistance to the clinical signs in birds after 2-3 weeks of age develops. Matured birds may experience a temporary drop in egg production (5-10%) but do not develop neurological symptoms, when infected.

Only young chicks show 40-60% morbidity with 25 to 50% mortality is seen in an average in the infected chick flocks. The chicks from immune breeder flocks show no or lower morbidity and mortality.

Postmortem lesions

No gross lesions are generally observed in the dead bird die of AE. Histo-pathological observations of the central nervous system reveal the non-purulent encephalomyelitis and ganglionitis of the dorsal root ganglia. Striking lesion observed is 'perivascular' infiltration of lymphocytes in all portions of the brain and spinal cord except in cerebellum. The infiltrated small tymphocytes pile up several layers to form impressive Cuffs. In mid-brain, two nuclei - n.routundus and n.ovoidalis show invariably loose 'microgliosis' which is considered to be pathognomic. Central 'Chromatolysis' (axonal reaction) of the neurons in the nuclei of the brain stem, especially of medulla oblongata is also a pathognomic lesion. The dying neurons with central chromatolysis are surrounded by satellite oligodentroglia and later, microglia phago-cytose the remains.

Diagnosis Isolation and identification of causative agent

Brain, pancreas and duodenum are reliable source for virus isolation by inoculation of these organ's suspensions in chicks or in SPF egg embryos. 6 days old SPF egg, embryos inoculated with yolk sac route and allowing them to hatch and observed the hatched out chicks for clinical sign of disease for 10 days post hatch will show typical clinical AE in them and histo-pathological exam of brain, medulla oblongata will show typical lesions of AE in them which are pathogenomic.

Chickens exposed to AEV develop antibodies that can be measured by standard Virus Neutralization (VN) test. Indirect Fluorescent Antibody (FA) and immune diffusion tests can be used for virus identification. Another method to detect immunity of a flock exposed to the AE infection is Embryo Susceptibility test (ES). Fertile eggs from the flocks to be tested are inoculated along with control SPF eggs for 6 days and are then inoculated via yolk sac route with 100 EID_{50} of 'egg adapted' calnek strain of AEV and the same are opened on 10 to 12 days post infection for observation of AE lesions. If 100% embryos are affected, the flock is considered as AE susceptible and if embryos less than 50% or 50% show AE lesions, the flock is considered to be 'Immunized' or 'Exposed' to AE infection.

Prevention and Control

Vaccination of the breeder stock is the only effective way to control or prevent the 'Clinical Disease' in the progeny commercial chicks as AE is clinically observed only during the 1st few weeks of chicks life and there is no time for preventive vaccination of these chicks for development of immunity before clinical manifestation of the disease.

The vaccination of breeder flock (with live AE vaccine) is possible only during the growing period between 8 weeks to 16 weeks in layer birds and between 8 weeks to 20 weeks in broiler birds because of the fact that unvaccinated chicks between 1st 8 weeks of life are fully susceptible for precipitation of 'Clinical AE', if inoculated with live AE vaccine virus and if they are vaccinated with live AE vaccine after the maturity of breeder chicks (i.e. 16 weeks in case of layer chicks and 20 weeks in case of broiler chicks), they can experience the 'egg drop' due to AE infection and their progeny can experience 'Clinical AE' after hatching within 1 to 3 weeks post hatch. However, the inactivated 'Calnek strain' (Embryo adapted) vaccine can be used in breeder birds even after maturity in prelay and mid-lay stage safely.

It is very important that the vaccine manufacturers should be very particular about 'Accidental embryo' adaptation of their vaccine seed virus used for live AE vaccine (Freeze dried) should not occur inadvertently. This is because of the fact that if embryo adaptation occurs due to 'over passaging' of the AE live vaccine seed virus, the capacity of live AE vaccine virus to multiply in duodenum and then produce vaccine viremia after oral administration of AE vaccine, is lost and hence, intraocular vaccine is unable to produce the desired level of immunity in the breeder chicks and if such vaccine is inoculated by 'wing web' route in pullets, it produces 'Clinical disease' in those pullets.

The accidental embryo adaption occurs in 'seed virus' stocks of vaccine manufacturers to the variable extent and it can be detected time to time by careful observation during monitoring of inoculated embryos used in production of vaccine for 'development of AE specific lesions of muscular dystrophy' in embryos which should not be present in normal live 'enterotropic' AE vaccine virus.

If such embryo lesions in few or more vaccine virus inoculated embryos are detected by vaccine manufacturer, they should eliminate such embryo adapted vaccine virus seed from vaccine manufacture or they should undertake few passages of such seed in susceptible chick inoculation through 'oral' route to eliminate 'Embryo adaptation' characteristic from their 'Seed virus'.

Avian Encephalomyelitis: Indian Scenario

There was no official record of AE in India until the end of the 20th century. However, sporadic 'Clinical incidences' of AE were observed by the author during his field investigations in early nineteen eighties in Vijaywada and Hyderabad (A.P.). The disease showed its appearance in North including Punjab, Haryana and Rajasthan poultry belts in the form of lameness problems in broiler commercial chicks in early age (within 3 weeks of age) during 1999 to 2000 followed by wide scale incidences in eastern U.P., Bihar, Chhattisgarh and West Bengal since 2002.

Ventri Biologicals division of VHL introduced their newly licensed AE live vaccine in 2002 which brought down the incidences of AE in above mentioned areas by the end of 2002.

However, renewed incidences of AE were recorded in these poultry belts on further wider scale by October, 2004. The investigations revealed that the Bio-security conditions on some integrator hatcheries were poor and the distances between replacement chick sheds and the grower bird sheds were inadequate leading to the transfer of live, AE vaccine virus from 10 week old grower vaccinated chicks to the younger unvaccinated chicks which precipitated AE clinical disease in them (Lameness and Ataxia).

This problem was resolved by use of experimental AE inactivated vaccine which could avoid the spread of live AE vaccine virus strain from the vaccinated chicks of 10 weeks age to the lower age group chicks and higher age group unvaccinated layer birds susceptible to AEV on multiage group poultry farms.

The author also came across the problem of 'embryo adaptation' due to inadvertent over passaging of vaccine seed virus of AE during his 'quality assurance' job in vaccine production unit while monitoring the titration of live AE vaccine Batch. He observed few embryos of AE vaccine titration, showing 'muscular dystrophy' lesions and subsequently the failure of potency test of that vaccine batch. He concluded that this failure of test is due to 'embryo adaption' of AE live vaccine seed virus, on the circumstantial evidence and hence the said 'vaccine seed' was given 2 SPF chick passages by oral route by his colleagues in R & D section and they could improve the seed virus to gain back the 'enterotropic' live AE vaccine seed status. This could avoid failure of the vaccine in the field.

Presently, AE vaccine in the field is officially available only in the 'live vaccine' form. However, it is necessary to make available the inactivated calnek type strain vaccine for use in adult pullets or the breeder birds as the integrator breeder farms are of multiple age groups and strict isolation of various age groups for avoiding cross contamination of AE live vaccine virus is next to impossible. This allows the precipitation of AE infections clinically on such farms in susceptible chicks/adult breeders. The only solution in such case is inactivated vaccine and hence, the need for its licensing.

Suggested Reading

Calnek, B.W., Taylor, P.J., Sevoian, M. (1960). Studies on avian encephalomyelitis. IV. Epizootiology. Avian Dis 4: 325-347.

Jungherr, E., Minard, E.L. (1942). The present status of avian encephalomyelitis. J Am Vet Med Assoc 100: 38-46.

Tannock, G.A. and Shafren, D.R. (1985). A rapid procedure for the purification of avian encephalomyelitis viruses. Avian Dis 29: 312-321.

Tannock, G.A. and Shafren, D.R. (1994). Avian encephalomyelitis: A review. Avian Pathol 23: 603-620.

Taylor, L.W., Lowry, D.C., Raggi, L.G. (1955). Effects of an outbreak of avian encephalomyelitis (epidemic tremor) in a breeding flock. Poult Sci. 34: 1036-1045.

❏❏❏

Chapter 14

Avian Infectious Coryza

Infectious Coryza (I.C.) is an acute bacterial, respiratory disease of chicken with economic significance, caused by *Haemophlius paragallinarum*. The early literature described this clinical syndrome as infectious group and the etiological agent of the same was eluded identification a number of years, as the disease were often masked in mixed infections. As early as 1920 Beach regarded that I.C. was a district clinical entity. De Blieck isolated the causative agent of coryza infection, i.e. contagious catarrh of the fowl, the name by which I.C. was known in these days. He described the causative agent as 'haemoglobinophilic bacterium' and named it as 'Bacillus haemoglolinophilus coryzae gallinarum' because of its growth requirement of 2 factors i.e. X (Hemin) and V- (Nicotinamide adenine dinucleotide (NAD). However, page found that all isolates recovered from I.C. cases require only one growth factor, namely V-factor (NAD). More recently V factor (NAD) independent isolates of H. paragallinarum have been recovered from I.C. in South Africa.

About the causative organism

Haemophlius paragallinarum is a gram negative non-motile becterium with short rods, cocco-bacillary or filamentous pleomorphic forms. Virulent strains of the organisms are capsulated. The organisms undergo degeneration within 48 to 60 hours, showing fragments and ill defined forms. The bacilli may occur singly, in pairs or as short chains.

Cultural requirements

The reduced from of NAD, i.e. hydrolysate of NAD (1.56-25 micro grammes/ml of medium) or its oxidized form (20-100 micro grammes/ml) is needed for growth on artificial medium for most of the isolates except for those from South African origin which are NAD independent. Sodium chloride (NaCl), 1 to 1.5% is essential for growth.

Some fastidious strains require 1% chicken serum for culturing. Brain-heart infusion, chicken meat infusion and tryptose agar with supplementation of NAD and x factor containing media are the best for obtaining profused growth of the organisms. The organisms require 5% carbon dioxide in the atmosphere or at least reduced oxygen tension or anaerobic condition for the growth with inoculation temperature range between 25⁰C to 45⁰C. Commonly they grow at 37⁰C temperature.

For the primary isolation of the organisms from Nasal sinus swab from infected bird, blood Agar plates streaked both horizontally and vertically with the culture loop from *'staphylococcus epidermidis'* isolate obtained from poultry bird's skin, before streaking of Nasal sinus swab are incubated under 5% CO_2 tension at 37⁰C–38⁰C in jar called 'secubator' is needed. Such blood agar plates will reveal 'Tiny dewdrop' like colonies upto 0.3 mm diameter as a 'satellite' growth around the staphylococcus epidermidis colonies. In obliquely transmitted light, these colonies are mucoid (smooth) iridescent but some colonies can be rough non-iridescent or of intermediate form.

The growth is catalase negative (no effervescence with hydrogen peroxide) and no fermentation of lactose, galactose and trehalose are some Bio-chemical characteristics which can differentiate haemophilus gallinaurm from Pasturella multoceda i.e. from I.C. and F.C. (Fowl cholera) organisms.

Antigenic structure and serotypes

Typing of *H. Paragallinarum* isolates below the species level has traditionally been done by serotyping. Page (1962) classified his 12 isolates of H. Paragallinarum in 3-serotypes using the plate agglutination test namely serovars A, B and C. Page serovar 'A' (strain 0083) and Serovar 'B' (strain 0222) are available today. However, his serovar 'C' strains were lost in the mid-1960's. Matsumoto and Yamamoto (1975) isolated 'Modesto' strain which was later on classified as serovar 'C' by Rimler *et al.* (1977), using cross protection test.

Based on Page's typing scheme and using photo agglutination test Germen isolates of I.C. were typed as serovar A and B (1973) Spanish strains classified as serovars A,B, and C (1986), strains from Australia, South Africa and Indonesia were typed as A and C.

It is also possible to use haemagglutination Inhibition (HI) test to serotype the *Haemophilus paragallinarum* strains under the page serotyping scheme. Chinese isolates were serotyped as serover A by Chen, *et al* (1993) and Argentina's serotypes (1993) and Brazilian serotypes as A, B and C by Blackall *et al.* (1994).

One more approach for classifying serotype of *Haemophlius paragallinarum* by page scheme is the use of monoclonal antibody panel developed by Blackall, *et al.* (1991) but poses problems as serovar B monoclonals are not available and some results with other serovars are confusing. The page scheme serovars and immunotype specificity have intimate co-relation and chicken vaccinated with bacteria of one serovar protects only against Homologus field serovar strains.

Kume, *et al.* (1983) developed an alternative serological classification scheme using H.I. test based on using gluteraldehyde-fixed chicken eryrthrocytes adsorbed with potassium thyo-cyanate treated bacterial isolates 'sonicated lysates' as antigen and known rabbit hyper immune sera against 3 serovars A,B and C. Page's serovars A, C and B were elevated to sero groups, I, II and III respectively and 7 serovars (HA-1 to HA-7) were recognized among the 3 sero-groups: 3 each for I and II and one for III. Many isolates that were found to be 'non-typeable' by original page scheme by agglutination test were easily typed using the Kume scheme. An 8th and 9th serovar have been recognized from Australia. The terminology of the Kume's scheme has recently been altered. Under this altered nomenclature, the 3-serotypes I, II & III are renamed as A, C and B, emphasing that Kume's serogrups A, B and C match page serovars A, B and C within each of the serogroups, the serovars and numbered sequencially allowing new serovars to be added in numerical order. Thus, the nine currently recognized Kume serovars are A-1, A-2, A-3, A-4, B-1, C-1, C-2, C-3 and C-4. This scheme is not used widely as it is technically demanding. As Kume's sero groups match page serovars, it is reasonable to assume that there is no cross-protection across Kume sero groups. C-1 & C-2 are cross protective and C-2 and C-4 are also cross protective.

Pathogenicity, pathogenesis and Epizootology

A range of factors have been associated with pathogenecity. Kume, *et al.* (1983) demonstrated that HA activity plays a key role in colonization of the organisms in both serovars A and C.

The capsule of *Haemophlius paragallinarum* has been shown to be associated with 'Colonisation' of the organisms and the lesions produced by the same in Infectious Coryza. Capsule also protects the organisms from bactericidal action of the normal serum. It is suggested that the capsule of the organism release a toxin which is responsible for the 'Coryza' disease.

It is shown that crude polysaccharide extracted from *Haemophlius paragallinarum* is toxic to chicken and it responsible for the toxic action produced after inoculation of the bacteria. However, its role during occurrence of the disease is unknown.

Chickens of all ages are susceptible for the disease (IC). Turkeys, pigeons, sparrows, ducks, crows are refractory for experimental infection. Chronic or healthy birds have been shown to be the main reservoir of the disease and its spread. 'Vertical transmission' of the disease is not demonstrated. The airborne route is shown to be responsible for spread of the disease on the isolated farms or from shed to shed on multiple age group farms.

Incubation period of the disease is very short which may often be 24 to 48 hours. The duration of the disease depends on the virulence of the organisms. In the absence of a concurrent infection, IC usually runs its course within 2-3 weeks but in the presence of existing mycoplasma galisepticum infection, the disease runs a prolonged course even up to 50 days.

About the symptoms and lesions of the disease

The birds show serous or mucous nasal discharge, facial oedama and conjunctivitis, the 'Unilateral' swelling below the eye is a usual manifestation of the disease. However, bilateral oedema can also be seen often. In males, swollen wattles may also be evident. Rales may be heard in birds with infection of the lower respiratory tract.

A 'Swollen head' like syndrome can be associated with broilers. Arthritis and septicaemia is observed in broilers and layers, in presence of other pathogens complicating the disease. Diarrhoea, decreased feed and water consumption, decreased egg production (10 to 40%) are the other manifestations of the disease, leading to high economic loss.

Highly toxigenic strains may cause high mortality even though generally mortality is low but morbidity is high. When complicated with other infections like infectious bronchitis, fowl pox, CRD and fowl cholera, IC is more severe and prolonged with increased mortality. Gross and H.P. lesions acute catarrhal inflammation of Nasal passage and sinuses, catarrhal conjunctivitis and subcutaneous oedema of face and wattles are quite common. However, rarely pneumonia and air sacculitis are observed.

Sloughing, disintegration and hyperplasia of mucosal and glandular epithelia with oedema and hyperemia with heterophillic infiltration in tunica propria of mucous membrance of nasal cavity and Nasal sinuses is invariable histopathological picture.

Diagnosis

I.C. may be diagnosed on the basis of a history of rapidly spreading disease with 'Coryza' is the main manifestation, combined with the isolation of a catalase negative, gram negative organisms showing satellitic growth on blood agar plate, streked with staphylococcus epidermidis culture. The typical Bio-chemical tests described previously can complete the final identification of the causative organism.

Another efficient diagnostic procedure is to inoculate the sinus exudates from the infected (suspected) bird or cultural isolate from such bird's nasal sinus into susceptible SPF chickens by intra-sinus route. The production of Coryza symptoms within 24-48 hours in the inoculated birds confirm the infectious coryza. If the number of organisms in the inoculums is small, it may take up to 1 week to reproduce the disease.

The serovar specific agglutination test was developed by adsorbing poly-saccharide antigens on the latex particles. This test is effective in detection of recent infection.

AGP test will detect antibodies 2 weeks post infection and up to at least 11 weeks post infection. The HI test detects serovar specific antibodies. Kato's strain 221 is used commonly as antigen for serovar A antibody detection. The bacterial cells haemagglutinate chicken erythrocytes. Trypsin treatment enhances this activity. The treatment of erythrocytes with gluterldehyde or formaldehyde increases the sensitivity of the test. For running the H.I. test, serial serum dilutions are prepared in tubes or wells in the plate and to these dilutions, trypsin treated bacterial cell antigen is added and mixtures in wells or tubes are incubated for neutralization of the antigen by serum antibodies.

Then, gluteraldehyde treated chicken erythrocyte suspension is added to the serum antigen mixture containing wells or tubes and again incubated. If the serum dilution has not neutralized the antigen, the same will haemagglutinate the treated RBCS and no button of RBCS will be formed at the bottom. However, if the serum dilution has neutralized the antigen, no haemagglutination will take place and the treated RBCS will form the button at the bottom of the Tube/well. Number of tubes/wells if show haemagglutination, the serum used is supposed to contain serum antibodies against serovar 'A' antigen and bird who's serum is used in the test is supposed to have suffered from IC, serovar A infection. While negative result indicates absence of exposure of the bird to IC serovar A infection.

The H.I. test is not possible directly as above in case of serovar C infection. However, additional treatment of potassium thiocyanate treatment to bacterial cells, then their sonication before addition of chicken serum and then gluteraldehyde treated chicken erythrocytes will make it to haemagglutinate for H.I. testing for serovar C antisera.

Treatment

Use of Sulphonamides and Sulpha + Trimethoprim and long acting Terramycin or Sulpha + Dihydrostreptomycin are some combinations of chemotherapeutic antibiotics of choice for treatment.

Preventive treatment

As the recovered birds from I.C. infection are carriers of the infection, replacement flocks from unknown sources should be avoided. Depopulation of infected flock without using any chemotherapy/antibiotic treatment is desirable to avoid recycling of the infection on the farm.

Immunization programme

Commercial I.C. vaccines containing serovars A,B and C immunogenic strains are used for prophylactic immunization programme. These vaccines are generally formaldehyde or thiomersal inactivated bacterins with aluminium hydroxide gel adjuvants or mineral oil adjuvants with arlacel and twin 80 emulsifiers, the former are supposed to give better immunization as per the literature. The commercial layer grower breeder flocks of 10 to 12 weeks age are vaccinated with oil adjuvanted/Alhydrogel adjuvanted bacterin followed by 2nd booster vaccination at 14 to 16 weeks age by intra-muscular route as the bacterial antigens are week antigens and need repeated vaccination for better immunity.

Indian Scenario of Infectious Coryza

During the early period of the establishment of poultry industry in India, in the late 1950's and 1960's, white leg horn and Rhode island birds on Govt. poultry farm used to show the cases of infectious 'Roupe' with typical unilateral swelling below the lower eyelids. No doubt they were the cases of infectious coryza but the then veterinarians were positivity unaware of existence of specific organisms, namely *Haemophilus para gallinarum* which are responsible for that problem. They were treating those cases with sulphadimidine and for prevention of these 'Roupe' cases, so called 'Roupe' mixture was being used in drinking water, once in a week routinely on Govt. poultry farms. This was the actual experience of the author (Dr. S.V. Pandit, 1963). We were also finding cases of 'Nutritional' Roupe with typical lesions of Vit. A deficiency in the crop of the affected birds. This may be predisposing cause of the coryza cases then, for which we were using 'lucern grass' which contain high quantum of 'provit A' i.e. xanthenes, as preventive treatment. In early eighties, Poultry Industry was posed with the recurrent problem of infectious coryza with unilateral eye swelling and facial swelling due to the mixed infection with I.B. in Hyderabad poultry belt. However, coryza vaccine was not available in those days. Even the European and British pharmacopoeia, was not having any monograph on I.C. vaccine.

Experimental Coryza Vaccine (inactivated) was developed by Ventri Biological Division of Venkateshwara Hatcheries during Mid-Eighties after isolation of causative agent namely H. Paragallinarum from the field cases and after extensive field trials, the commercial licensed oil adjuvanted I.C. vaccine (inactivated) was launched by them in 1987. Combined fowl cholera and Infectious Coryza vaccine was also made available in 1993 for use as booster vaccination to avoid handling stress of 2 separate vaccines for these 2 diseases (FC and IC). Dr. Pat Blackall of Animal Research Institute, Queensland, Austerlia visited India in, April, 1999 and helped Ventri Biological Division of VHL to develop typing facilities for *Haemophlius paragallinarum* which enabled them to include known immunogenic typed strains, namely A and C serovars of cume, in their coryza vaccine.

However, it was observed that in spite of use of serovars A and C containing I.C. vaccine(s), the outbreaks of Coryza were still observed time to time in various parts of Andhra (Hyderabad, Anakapalli, Guntur, Ananparthi) and Barwala, Panipat, Sonepart, Jind, etc. of Punjab and Haryana. My personal discussions with Dr. Blackall revealed that possibility of immune suppression due to usage of hot IBD vaccines, VVIBD infection itself, CAA and Reo Viruses as well as IBH/HPS adenoviruses, VVMD infections precipitating the IC infection cannot be ruled out.

It seems that due to these immune suppressive problems, the affecting age groups of normal I.C. infection which was supposed to be 12 to 16 weeks has now come down to 4 to 8 weeks. This has resulted into difficulty in I.C. vaccination time. In general, I.C. vaccination is recommended by the manufactures at 10 to 12 weeks followed by booster vaccination at 13 to 16 weeks. But now the disease is observed at 8th to 9th week, then there is no proper age group available for 1st vaccination. The scope for recommendation of vaccination is still unlimited.

Suggested Reading

Blackall, P.J., Y.Z. Zheng, T. Yamaguchi, Y. Iritani, and Rogers, D.G. (1991). Evaluation of a panel of monoclonal antibodies in the subtyping of Haemophilus paragallinarum. Avian Dis. 35: 955–959.

Blackall, P.J., Silva, E.N., Yamaguchi, Y. and Iritani, Y. (1994). Characterization of isolates of avian haemophili from Brazil. Avian Dis. 38: 269–274.

Kume, K., A. Sawata, Nakai, T. and Matsumoto, M. (1983). Serological classification of Haemophilus paragallinarum with a hemagglutinin system. J. Clin. Microbiol. 17: 958–964.

Matsumoto, M. and Yamamoto, R.A. (1975). Protective quality of an aluminium-hydroxide-adsorbed broth bacterin against infectious coryza. Am. J. Vet. Res., 36: 579-582.

Page, L.A. (1962). Haemophilus infection in chickens. 1. Characteristics of 12 Haemophilus isolates recovered from diseased chickens. Am. J. Vet Res., 23: 85-95.

Rimler, R.B., Shotts, E.B. and Davis, R.B. (1975). A growth medium for the production of a bacterin for immunization against infectious coryza. Avian Dis., 19: 318-322.

Chapter 15

Avian Spirochetosis

Avian spirochaetosis is a tick-borne acute septicaemic disease of birds caused by spiral form bacteria called as *Borrelia anseria*, characterized by marked illness, variable morbidity and high mortality.

Even though Avian spirochaeate is closely related to Borrelia species, namely *B. burgdorferi* which share common flagellar antigens and which produces human Lyme disease, it has no public health importance (Walker, *et al.*, 1989).

History, Incidence and Distribution

Avian spirochaetosis was first recorded in Russia by Sakharoff (1891) in geese while the first description of fowl spirochactosis is found from Brazil in 1903, wherein role of fowl ticks as primary vector was identified (Smit, H.F., 1996 – personal communication mentioned by H.J. Barness (author of 'Spirochactosis' in 'Diseases of Poultry' book). This disease is first described in USA amongst turkeys in California, in 1946. Recently, spirochaetosis was diagnosed in game chickens in California (Cooper and Bickford, 1993).

The disease occurs worldwide but most frequently in tropical and subtropical warm and humid regions. Sporadic outbreaks of relatively mild disease occurs in the South-western United States.

About the Causative Organism

Borrelia anserine belongs to the order *Spirochactales* and family *Spirochactaceae* of bacteria. It is a highly motile helical bacterium with 5 to 8 spirals. It can pass through 0.45 micron. It has 15-22 flagella which are in the periplasmic space beneath the outer cell membranes and are attached sub terminally near the ends of and overlap (30-44 flagella) at the middle of the spirochete. It morphologically differs from 'treponemes' and 'leptospires' and hence, stain readily with ordinary aniline dyes. It is usually stained by Romanowasky type stains like leishman or Giemsa stains or by silver impregnation method.

The organism can be easily identified in wet smears of blood or tissue suspensions under the phase contrast microscope or by dark-field microscope. Spirochactes are unable to grow on ordinary bacteriological media but can be grown successfully in Barbour stoenner Kelly medium with difficulty and are lost after 10-12 passages. The organisms are microaerophilic and reproduce by binary fission. They produce acid from glucose.

The spirochetes can be serially passaged from one bird to another by transmission of infected blood. They can also be passaged in chicken embryos by yolk sac route inoculation. They are more numerous in liver, blood and membranes of the infected egg embryo but only few organisms are seen in extra embryonic fluids, uncontaminated by blood. They are very fragile and are not resistant to ordinary disinfectants. They can survive in infected chicken carcasses at 0°C for one month and they can be stored in serum for 3-4 weeks at + 4°C temperature in refrigerator.

The strains can be preserved in -70°C deep freezer or in liquid nitrogen, when frozen with 10-15% glycerol or dimethyl sulphoxide (DMSO). Multiple serotypes exist in nature which may or may not cross protect each other in birds. Strains also differ in virulence (Cooper, *et al.*, 1993) but no distinct serotyping scheme is evolved for this pathogen.

Pathogenesis and epizootology

Chickens, turkeys, ducks, geese and canaries have been naturally infected with this organism. Local breeds of chicken are more resistant to infection than commercial birds. Pigeons and guinea fowl are relatively resistant to infection.

The infectious organisms can be transmitted by blood, excreta and tissues of recently infected or dead birds to the susceptible or injection of blood or droppings via contaminated feed and water or use of syringe or needless contaminated with infected blood or tissues can transmit the disease to susceptible birds coming in contact with it/got injected with it.

Mosquitoes, biting arthropods including fowl mites are capable of transmitting the disease. Soft ticks belonging to genus Argus is the most important transmitter and the reservoir of the infective organisms. B. anserina cannot survive for long time in birds or outside in environment and it only survives and multiplies in tick for its continued existence. All Argus species cannot carry infection for long time but in Argus persicus, it survives for longest time.

After feeding on heavily infected chicken by *A. persicus*, spirochactes are found in good numbers in the gut of the human tick initially, decline in numbers in the next week and becomes immobile by 15-20 days and die by 20 days. However, some spirochactes penetrate the gut wall within 2 hours of feeding and are then present in haemolymph where they multiply during next 7 days. Then, they are found in tissues of ticks including salivary glands, gonads, and central nervous tissue mass, where they survive for about 2 months. The spirochactes survive even moulting of tick larval stages to adults and are also transferred to next generation by transovarian route. Infection of rat can be as high as 100%.

The ticks become infective 6-7 days after biting a host and can remain infective upto 488 days (Knowles, *et al.*, 1932). Larval ticks can remain attached to the birds and can feed for 4-5 days in contrast to the nymphs and adults which show nocturnal habit for temporary attachment to the host during night and hiding in cracks and crevices in the poultry premises during daytime, thus escaping the notice of the workers on the farm. The tick activity increases during warmer and humid summer and the organisms develop most rapidly and hence, outbreaks are more frequent in summer season. Birds become infected from saliva of ticks introduced, when bitten or by ingesting infected ticks or ova by the birds. Recovered birds are not carriers of the infection as spirochactes disappear from tissues of them after recovery.

About the disease

Incubation period of the disease varies from 3 to 12 days depending upon how organisms have entered the body and by which route. After IV route entry, there can be 100% infection and mortality.

The infected birds are visibly sick, with cyanosis of comb & wattles, ruffled feathers, droppy palor, huddled up appearance and greenish diarrhoea. The birds can be inactive and anorexic. Body temperature can abruptly rise upto 30^{0}C and in turkeys it may rise even upto 43^{0}C. Body weight is lost rapidly. Birds may develop paresis or paralysis in late stages, birds becoming confused. Body temperature can be subnormal at the end.

The birds may develop severe anaemia, marked reduction in erythrocytic numbers, PCV and haemoglobin. Peak of anaemia occurs when spiro organisms disappear from blood circulation. Morbidity and mortality can be variable from 1-2% to 100%. It can be very high in previously unexposed flocks but in closed flocks with chronic exposure, the birds become immune and resistant due to the presence of maternal immunity and show low rate of morbidity and mortality.

Gross lesions are characterized by enlargement of spleen with mottled surface. The liver may also be enlarged and contain small haemorrhages and pale foci, occasional marginal infarcts of liver can also be evident. Kidneys are also swollen with pale uratic deposits. Intestinal contents can be green and mucoid, hemorrhages can be observed at proventricular junction. Mild fibrinous pericarditis may be present.

Diagnosis

Clinical diagnosis of spirochactosis can be made by observation of typical clinical symptoms and lesions described above and demonstration of spirochactes in blood and infected organ smears after staining with Giemsa or Leishman stain or by Fontana's silver impregnation stain.

Confirmation of spirochactosis needs demonstration of either organisms or their antigens during clinical illness. The stained smears when observed under light microscope reveal typical spiral structure of the organism. However, the observation of wet drop preparation of fluid blood or tissue suspension under phase contrast microscope or dark field illumination can show the floating and swimming spiral organisms typically. The infected blood/tissue suspension can be inoculated on 6 days old SPF egg embryos by yolk sac route in case the organisms are not sufficiently present in direct smears and the examination of the infected egg embryo's liver or spleen tissue will show typical spirochetes in the stained tissue smear.

Serological Diagnosis

Serum plate agglutination test, slide agglutination and immobilization test, agar gel precipitin test and indirect fluorescent antibody test are the different serological tests which can be performed on paired sera samples at infectious and recovery stages for demonstration of rising antibody titres for sero-confirmation of the disease.

Differential Diagnosis

Acute septicacmic diseases like fowl typhoid, fowl cholera and coli-septicaemia and viral infections like NDV, AI and marek's disease is required to be eliminated before coming to final diagnosis as spleenomegali with mottling and liver and kidney swelling can be present in many of above diseases. Greenish diarrhoea and pro-ventricular lesions in NDV and A.I. also can confuse with spirochactasis. The serological and histopath examination can be done for differential diagnosis.

Treatment (Theraputic)

Arsenic preparations and antibiotics including penicillin, tetracyclines, terramycin, etc. are highly effective for curative effect.

Prevention and control

Depopulation of houses and burning of cracks and crevises using suitable gas or kerosin tourch burners for eradication of the fowl tick population is practiced for control of transmission of spirochactes through vectors. Larval stages of ticks can be controlled by dipping birds in 0.5% malathione. Malathione or gamaxine dusting of birds is also useful for this purpose. High pressure spraying of the house and environment, paying particular attention to cracks, crevises and places where ticks hide, with 3% Malathion at monthly intervals can keep tick population at the low level. Authors have came across an outbreak in local farm, wherein wooden perches were used in economic growers. Hence, use of wooden material is better avoided. Tick proof roosters by placing in oil filled containers help in reaching of infected ticks up to the birds while resting.

Immunization

Vaccines prepared from lysates of blood, tissues or embryos infected with B.anserina, inactivated with formaldehyde or phenol and adjuvanted with oil (mineral oil with arlacel and tween 80 as emulsifying agents) are useful for prolonged prevention of the disease. Use of polyvalent vaccine with multiple serotypes is better than monovalent strain vaccines need to be prepared using autogenous strains for specific areas to get better homologous immunity. Deliberate infection, followed by antibiotic treatment 3 days later has also been used to induce immunity.

Indian Scenario regarding Avian Spirochaactosis (Tick fever)

Avian spirochactosis (Tick fever) was prevalent in India, in early forties. Kapur (1940) has described transmission of spirochactosis through agents other than ticks *A. persicus* in those days. Tick borne spirochactosis infection was rampant on Govt. and Private Poultry farms during nineteen fifties and sixties and even the infection was prevalent in village backyard poultry in those days in sporadic form, wherever soft ticks existed with nocturnal habbit of biting poultry birds and hiding in cracks and crevices of poultry house flooring and perches and wooden feeder and waterers since old days.

However, practice of flame gunning of cracks and crevices on the floorings, cages and feeders/waterers could effectively bring down this infection in nineteen seventies and eighties onwards. This could improve poultry production on Govt. and private poultry farms significantly. Mehta and Muley (1969) have described use of spirochactosis vaccine produced from 'Jabalpur Strain' of *B. gallinarum* with high efficacy. Rao (1958) had written an exhaustive review on fowl spirochactosis in India. Soni and Joshi. (1980) have written a note on strain variation between 'Akola' and 'Jabalpur' strains on Avian spirochactosis.

Verma and Mallick (1968) have described diagnosis of spirochactosis by agar gel diffusion test and Wadalkar, *et al.* (1982) has given an account of use of FAT for its diagnosis. State Veterinary Biological production units (e.g. IVBP, Pune, IVPM, Ranipat, B.P. Division Mhow and Jabalpur) produced inactivated wet Avian spirochactosis vaccines using formalized blood from spirochactosis infected birds and kept their strains of spirochactes by blood to blood passage in poultry birds for 'Seed bank'. These vaccines were used on limited scale in local states.

However, Ventri Biological Division of Venkateshwara Hatcheries, Pune produced oil adjuvanted formalin inactivated vaccine keeping their 'Seed stock' of spirochetes preserved in Liquid nitrogen, using glycerol or dimethyl sulphoxide (DAMSO) as cryo-preservative. This vaccine was introduced by them in the field, in 1990 and is being presently in north and central India upto date (2007), wherever sporadic incidences of spirochactasis still occur.

Suggested Reading

Cooper, G.L and Bickford, A.A. (1993).Spirochetosis in California game chicken. Avian dis, 7: 1176-1171.

Kapur, H.R. (1940). Transmission of Spirochetosis through agent other than argas persicus. Indian. J. Vet. Sci. Anim. Husb, 10: 354-366 cited by Barnes, H.J. (1997). In. Disease of poultry 10 edition edited by B.W. Calnek with H. JohnBarnes, C.W.; Beard, I.R. McDougland Y.M. Saif. Iowa state University press Ames, Iowa USA (1997).

Knowles, R.; Das Gupta, B.M and Basu, B.C. (1932). Studies on avian spirochetosis. Indian Med. Res. Mem. 22: 100-113.

Mehta, M.L. and Muley, A.R. (1968). *In vitro* agglutination and immobilization lysis for typing antigenically different strains of borrelia gallinarum. Indian. Vet. J., 45: 1059.

Rao, S.B.V. (1958). Spirochetosis in poultry. Indian Council of Agricultural Research, New Delhi, India. Research series No. 18.

Sakharoff, M.N. (1891). Spirochete anserina *et al* septicemia des OIE Ann Inst Pastuer 5: 564-566. Cited by Barnes, H.J. (1997). In B.W. Calnek with disease of poultry 10 edition edited by; McDougland Y.M. Saif. Iowa, H. JohnBarnes, C.W.; Beard, I.R. state University press Ames, Iowa, USA (1997).

Soni, J.L. and Joshi, A.G. (1980). A note in strain variation in Akola and Jabalpur strains of Borrelia anserina. Zlbl. Vet. Med. (B)27: 70-72.

Verma, K.G. and Malik, B.S. (1968). Diagnosis of poultry by slide agglutination test. Curr Sci 37: 170.

Walker, R.L.; Greene, R.T.; Nicholson, W.L. and Levine, J.F. (1989). Shared flagellar Epitopes of Borrelia burgdorferi and Borrelia anserina. Vet. Microbiology. 19: 361-371.

❑❑❑

Chapter 16

Salmonella Infections of Poultry Origin

Infections with bacteria of the genus *Salmonella* are responsible for a variety of acute and chronic diseases in poultry and comprise one of the most important reservoirs of salmonellae that can be transmitted through the food chain to humans. Isolation of salmonellae are reported more often from poultry and poultry products than from any other animal species.

The genus *Salmonella* of the family *Enterobacteriacae* is named after USDA veterinarian and bacteriologist Daniel E. Salmon and it consists of more than 2300 serologically distinct variants (serotypes). All *Salmonellae* can be grouped into only 5 subgenera which are often epidemiologically relevant.

Poultry salmonellae can be grouped into 3 categories, namely: 1) Generally host specific salmonellae (*S. Pullorum and S. gallinarum*) for avian species, which produce specific poultry diseases, including pullorum disease also called Bacillary White Diarrhoea (BWD) in chicks and Fowl Typhoid (FT) in matured birds, 2) Motile *salmonella* serotypes, collectively called as 'Paratyphorid salmonellae' which cause food borne disease in humans. They comprise of a group of more than 2300 sero-groups but only 10% out of these sero-groups are identified to be carried by poultry and produce significant disease losses in young chickens only but more significantly they are responsible for 'food poisoning' in humans through the use of contaminated poultry products (meat and eggs). The most important representative serotypes of 'Para-typhoid group' from poultry origin are salmonella entertidis and salmonella typhimurium. 3) Group of serotypes of subgenus Arizonne is bio-chemically distinct and causes a disease that is not clinically distinguishable from other salmonella infections. 'Arizonosis' is of particular economic significance in Turkeys. As Turkeys are not significantly reared in India, this group in this chapter is not dealt with.

The poultry salmonella problem has attained significant importance in recent years. Previously in the beginning of poultry industry in India, primary action for controlling salmonella infections in poultry was to reduce disease losses. Today public health concerns, political pressures and consumer's demands have increasingly made prevention of Food borne transmission of disease to humans an urgent priority for poultry producers.

Pullorum disease and fowl typhoid have been effectively dealt within USA and other developed countries by a strategy of testing and eradication. However, the strategy for controlling paratyphoid (PT) *Salmonellae* have to be correspondingly 'broader' than that applied for 'avian adapted' serotypes as PT salmonellae are not host specific. They are nearly ubiquitous in domestic animals, wild animals and humans and poultry trade becoming 'global' it has created new and more complex opportunities for the 'spread' of salmonellae. The combined application of number of control measures, including: 1) Testing programs, 2) Production of salmonellae Free feed, 3) Elimination of biological vectors (Rats, Mice, Squirrels), 4) Effective cleaning and disinfection of poultry houses and 5) Prophylactic treatment of poultry birds (vaccination measures, probiotic and antibiotic treatment) for 'reduction though' 'not elimination' of shedding of salmonellae by the infected / carrier birds may be necessary to achieve the tangible results in overall reduction of 'paratyphoid' salmonellae.

Pullorum disease and fowl typhoid

Pullorum disease (PD) and fowl typhoid (FT) have many similarities in terms of history, clinical signs, epizootology, lesions and control/eradication measures.

Pullorum disease (PD) is caused by *Salmonella pullorum* and fowl typhoid is caused by *Salmonella galinarum*. Both the diseases cause septicaemia and primarily affect chickens and turkeys and are transmitted through the eggs by trans-ovarian infection. They are highly host adapted and are considered as the same species (salmonella pullorum - galinarum) in Europe and some other countries. Both FT and PD produce rare infections in human and are of little public health importance. Etiological agent of PD was described by Retter in 1899. It was widespread in USA and many other countries throughout the world even upto 1932, with mortality ranging upto 100%, seriously threatening the chicken industry. Egg born transmission of PD was proved between 1900 and 1910. The application of Tube agglutination test for detection of carriers of the organisms was described in 1913. Slide agglutination test using whole blood and stained antigen was developed in 1931 which is used widely because of its simplicity.

The National Poultry Improvement Plan (NPIP) was established in USA by state agencies co-operating with USDA was established in 1935 designed in part to control PD in chicken. National Turkeys Improvement Plan (NTIP) on the lines of NPIP was established in 1943, in USA. Series of modifications in these 2 plans over the years have helped in eradication of PD in commercial poultry in USA by 1980. However, series of outbreaks occurred in 1990-91 and 1992. Thereafter, no outbreaks of PD are officially reported in USA in commercial poultry but the disease still occurs in backyard poultry.

Fowl Typhoid (FT) is closely related to PD and is caused by salmonella gallinarum, first recognized in 1888 but the name FT was applied in 1902. It was first recognized in USA but later on soon detected in Germany and Netherlands. Control of FT was included in NPIP of USDA in 1954 which is the main reason for the near eradication of FT in commercial poultry in USA with low incidence in all poultry.

There are low incidences of FT in Canada, United States and several European countries. Outbreaks of FT have been recorded in Denmark, in 1994. Dramatic increase in FT incidence was reported from Mexico, Central and South America and Africa in 1964, 1984, 1988 respectively.

Etiology of PD and FT

S. pullorum and *S. gallinarum* are members of family *Enterobacteriacae* and are highly host-adapted to poultry. They are non-motile, belonging to serogroup 'D' of 'Kauffman white schema'. They are now listed as '*S. gallinarum pullorum*'. Both Salmonellae are shown by mubbiloans enzyme electrophoresis and chromosomal genotypic diversity that they are 'monophyletic' while *S. enteritidis* is a 'Polyphyletic' serotype and all these 3 are closely related.

The organisms are gram negative, non-sporogenic, non-motile and facultative anaerobic. They are slender rods occurring singly but occasionally two or more rods are found.

They grow readily on beef agar or broth or other nutrient media aerobically/facultative anaerobically at 37^{0}C. They grow in selective enrichment media like selenite broth or tetrathyonate broth and differential solid media, such as Mac Conkey, bismuth sulphite and brilliant green agars. S. pullorum grows slower than S. gallinarum.

Both *S. pullorum* and *S. gallinarum* ferment arabinose, Dextrose, gal-lactose, mannitol, mannose and xylose but do not ferment lactose, sucrose and salicin.

S. gallinarum ferments usually dulcitol and maltose while *S. pullorum* does not ferment dulcitol and occasionally ferments maltose (generally does not ferment maltose). Major difference is shown by using Ribotyping (enzyme ECORI has been shown to be important tool to differentiate between S. pullorum and S. gallinarum.

Antigenic structure

Both *S. pullorum* and *S. gallinarum* possess the O antigens 1, 9 and 12. Sometimes, variation occurs in antigen 12 in case of *S. pullorum* but this does not happen in *S. gallinarum*. The antigenic composition of *S. pullorum* was shown to be 9,12,12_2,12_3, the variation involved antigens 12_2,and 12_3, standard strain of S. pullorum contain large amount of 12_3 and very small amount of 12_2 but variant strains content of these 2 antigens is 'reversed'.

Early reports from USA indicated as many as one-third of S. pullorum isolates were of 'variant' type but by 1950 only 13% of total isolates were of that type, which was a result of extensive use of polyvalent testing antigens.

Tests to differentiate standard, intermediate and variant types of *S. pullorum* using 'ammonium sulphate precipitation test' is described by Williams. (1953). Phage typing of *S. pullorum* can be used for identification of type of epidemiological investigation and genetic studies (Tsubokura. 1965 and 1966 and Christensen, *et al.*, 1992 respectively). Endotoxins from *S. gallinarum* have been shown to cause clinical illness within few house of intravenous inoculation in chicks.

It is shown that particular genes are responsible for efficient adherence and entry of various salmonellae into cultured epithelial cells. Plasmid with 8.5 kb size plays a role in virulence of both S. pullorum and S. gallinarum.

Age of Host commonly infected

PD mortality is usually confined to the first 2-3 weeks of age and certain percentage of chickens that survive the initial infection in early chick age become 'Carriers' with or without the presence of lesions.

FT is frequently referred to as a disease of adult birds. However, there are many reports of high mortality in young chickens, which can reach even upto 26%.

Transmission of the disease

Both PD and FT can be transmitted by several ways. The infected 'reactor and carrier' bird perpetuates and spreads the infection through infected hatching eggs. Birds may infect not only their own generation but also succeeding generation through egg transmission. This can result from contamination of ovum following ovulation but localization of *S. pullorum* or *S. gallinarum* in the ovules before ovulation is also likely and constitutes the chief mode of transmission. Shell penetration and feed contamination of S. pullorum is reported but is of minor importance.

Contact transmission of infected chicks or pullets is an important route of dissemination of both the pathogens. Mortality by this way upto 60.9% is reported. Faecal contamination of feed as a route of the transmission of the diease is also important. Visitors and traders are also incriminated as source of infection.

Clinical Disease

In case of PD, the chicks hatched from infected eggs are found dead within short period after hatching. The infected chicks may show weakness, loss of appetite poor growth and adherence of chalky white material to the vent. Death may soon fallow. In some cases disease is seen only after 5 to 10 days after hatching. The peak of mortality is generally occurring in 2nd and 3rd weak of life. The birds huddle together with droopy wings and distorted body appearance. Extensive lung affection may cause laboured breathing. Survivors show retarded growth and poor feathering. The survivors become carriers of the disease. Blindness and swelling of humero-radial and ulner articulation has been described. Sinovitis and swelling of hock joints is also observed.

In adult birds, generally of FT and in few instances PD, the chickens show ruffled feathers, shrunken combs, drop in egg production, decreased fertility and diminished hatchability, depending upon severity of infection. Death may occur in 4 days of exposure to 5-10 days of infection. Anorexia, diarrhoea, depression and dehydration are prominent symptoms. Mortality is variable from 0 to 100%, depending on bird's susceptibility, age, nutrition of the flock, etc. Mortality up to 93% due to FT in chicks is also reported.

Gross lesions

In acute cases of chicks, enlarged and congested liver, spleen and kidneys with white necrotic foci on liver can be seen. Unabsorbed yolk sacs may be observed in chicks. Whitish nodules in the lungs and cardiac muscle can be observed in some cases. The cardiac nodules may result in chronic passive congestion of heart muscles leading to distortion of heart and ascitis. In adult birds, small nodular or regressing ovarian follicles can be found. Lesions found in chronic carrier hens, however, are a few mis-shapen, discoloured cystic ova giving 'Coliflower' like appearance with pedunculated ova. Often, the oviduct contains caseous exudates in lumen. Abdominal ovulation may occur with oviduct impaction, leading to extensive 'egg peritonitis'. Ascitis may also develop.

Pericarditis with thickened opaque pericardial sac and pericardial fluid may also be evident. In males testicals may have white foci or nodules. Occasional caseous granulomas can be found in lungs and air sacs.

Histopathological lesions

Multifocal Necrosis of heptocytes with accumulation of fibrin and infiltration of heterophils in liver are seen. Periportal infiltration of heterophils mixed with few lymphocytes and plasma cells in glyson's capsules are also observed in liver.

In chronic cases, with large nodules in heart, the liver will have chronic passive congestion with interstitial fibrosis. In the heart, infiltration of heterophils mixed with lymphocytes and plasma cells is seen. In later stages, histocytic type fairly large cells with irregular vascular nuclei and faintly staining foamy eosinophilic cytoplasm are seen.

Diagnosis

Diagnosis of PD and FT can be done by isolation of respective salmonella organisms from visceral organs and heart blood using selective selenite broth and subsequent streaking of the same after incubation (24 hrs) on Mac Conkey agar showing non-lactose fermenting colonies. Typical gramme negative rods in singles, in the smears from colonies from Mac Ckonkey's agar plates and agglutination of loopful of organisms suspended in 'Saline drop' on glass slide by addition of known hyper-immune serum against *S. Pullorum/gallinarum* will confirm the practical diagnosis. The confirmative diagnosis is possible by studying the bio-chemical tests described previously.

Prevention and Control

It is now established fact that chicken flocks can be developed and maintained free of PD and FT by adhering to well defined procedure laid down by 'NPIP' programme of USDA. These procedures include basic managemental procedures and well organized PD/FT testing programme. It is mandatory that only eggs from flocks known to be free from PD/FT be introduced into hatchery. The following management procedures should be broadly applied:

1. Chicks and poults should be obtained from sources free of PD & FT.
2. No mixing of pullorum free and typhoid free stocks with other poultry or confined birds not known to be free from PD & FT.
3. Chicks should be placed in an environment that can be cleaned and sanitized to eliminate any residential salmonellae from previous flocks.
4. Chicks and poults should receive pelletized crumbled feed to minimize the introduction of S. Pullorum/Gallinarum or other salmonellae through contaminated feed ingredients. Use of feed ingredients free of salmonellae is highly desirable.
5. Introduction of salmonellae from outside sources must be minimized by use of a sound bio-security programme.
6. Free flying birds (supposed to be carriers of salmonellae) should not be allowed to reach the bird sheds by making them bird proof.

7. Rats, mice, rabbits, cats, dogs and pests which are carriers of salmonellae should be kept away from bird sheds by using 'Rodent proof skirting' around them.
8. Insect control against flies, poultry mites and lesser mealworms (bittles) should be undertaken using proper pest control treatments.
9. Potable drinking water duly chlorinated or sanitizer treated should be used in poultry sheds to avoid salmonella entry through drinking water
10. Use of foot baths, restricted foot ware and clothing to be provided.
11. Proper disposal of dead birds by burning or burial.

Elimination of carrier birds

NPIP control programme envisages 2 or 3 consecutive re-tests of the poultry flocks using quick whole blood agglutination test against salmonella pullorum gallinarum standard plate test antigen to clear off the possible 'Salmonella reactors' from the farm/shed. It is necessary that 2 consecutive tests should be negative for salmonella reactors to declare the flock as 'Salmonella free'. The following steps to be undertaken to avoid 'reinfection' during testing prgoramme:

1. The 'Positive Reactors' should be removed from the tested flock immediately after the test and should be destroyed and disposed off properly or taken to the laboratory away from 'flocks' for isolation of salmonellae for confirmation.
2. The tested negative flock should be transferred to the new duly disinfected shed and kept there until completion of the next test.
3. The original shed of the birds, after emptying of tested flocks, should be thoroughly disinfected for total removal of salmonella infection, before re-using it for bringing back the flock after retest (2nd test).
4. Retesting (2nd test) should be carried out 3 to 4 weeks after the 1st test and positive reactors found, if any, should be destroyed and discarded by proper disposal. The retested birds may be brought back to the original disinfected shed.
5. The above steps 1 to 4 to be repeated until 2 consecutive re-tests are found negative for salmonella reactors.

6. Doubtful reactors should not be mixed with original flock but to be kept 'Segregated' and re-tested after 3-4 weeks and if found 'negative', they may be mixed with original flock and if confirmed as 'Positive' reactors, they should be destroyed and cultured for further confirmation.
7. Non-pullorum/gallinarum reactors are non-specific reactors which are found 'positive' on testing but from which no 'salmonella pullorum/gallinarum can be isolated. These reactions may be due to birds exposure to staphylococcus epidermidis or micrococcus or *E. coli* or proteus and other similar organisms. These reactions can also be due to salmonellae other than pullorum gallinarum group. But such reactors should not be allowed to remain in 'Salmonella free' flock.

Area Eradication Programme

The following are the essentials for eradication of salmonella pullorum gallinarum from an area:

1. PD and F.T. should be mandatory reportable diseases.
2. Outbreaks must be placed under quarantine and infected flocks marketed under supervision.
3. All reports to be investigated by authorized state or federal official.
4. Importation of eggs and poultry should be only from sources certified to be free from salmonella infection.
5. Flocks going to public exhibition should be free from salmonella.
6. Total participation of poultry breeding flocks and hatcheries must be required in a pullorum typhoid control programme, such as NPIP or equivalent.

Preventive vaccines and vaccinations

As PD has been mostly eradicated from commercial flocks over the long years back, nothing much is known or done for preventive vaccine development for PD. However, FT continues to be still global problem. Vaccine development work against FT is going on in various parts of the world. However, there is no federally licensed FT bacterin (inactivated) in USA and live vaccines used in other parts of the world are not licensed in USA.

With rise in FT problems all over the world, studies on use of 9 R strain as live oral or injectable vaccine, with or without oil adjuvants have been reported with variable results (Gupta, *et al.* 1976 and Silva, *et al* 1981). Similarly, outer membrane proteins (OMP) from S. gallinarum have been reported to offer better protection than 9R live vaccine in terms of clearance of pathogenic strain from internal organs. (Bouzouback and Nagraja K.V., *et al.*, 1987).

More recently, immunization against F.T. by use of mutant strains of S. gallinarum and a virulence plasmid-cured derivative of S. gallinarum appears to be promising in protecting birds challenged with S. gallinarum (Barrow, P.A. 1990 and 1992 and griffin H.G., *et al.*, 1993).

Paratyphoid Infections of Poultry

As mentioned in the beginning of this chapter, the paratyphoid infections (PT infections), other than asymptomatic intestinal carriage, continue to cause significant disease losses in young poultry. In addition to this, PT salmonellae have been the subject of intensified interest as agents of food borne disease transmission to humans. Poultry products are consistently identified as important source of salmonellae that cause illness in humans and more than 1/3 rd of food borne salmonellosis outbreaks in humans in USA between 1983 and 1987 were associated with poultry meat or eggs (Tauxe, R.V. 1991).

Most commonly identified serotypes of PT salmonellae between July, 1990 to June, 1993 were *S. heidelberg, S. entertidis, S. saintpaul* and *S. typhimurium*, both from poultry and human in USA. Because of the unique epidemiological association of *S.enteritidis* with disease transmission via contaminated eggs to human beings its specific prevalence has gained considerable importance in recent years. It was noticed that only 10% incidence of *S.enteritidis* through contaminated eggs in human beings in 1979 has increased to 47% in 1987 in USA and Europe.

Etiology : Various motile and non-host adapted serotypes of subgenus 1 out of total 5 biochemically distinct subgenera, are referred to as PT salmonellae. PT salmonellae are also gram negative rods similar in description to salmonella pullorum gallinarium (typhoid group), but unlike Salmonella Pullorum gallinarum which are non-motile, PT salmonellae are motile with peritricous flagella and their colonies are found with smooth edges, slightly raised and glistening.

Their nutritional requirements are similar to typhoid group. They ferment glucose (acid + gas) dulcitol, maintol, maltose but do not ferment lactose, sucrose and salicin.

Paratyphoid salmonellae differ from *S. pullorum* by the fact that *S. pullorum* cannot ferment dulcitol.

Antigenic structure : The antigenic classification of salmonellae is based on both somatic and flagellar antigens.

The somatic 'O' antigens are determined by polysaccharides associated with the body of the organism and are identified by 'Arabic' numbers. Serogroups (designated with upper case letters) of salmonellae are defined by particular somatic antigens that are unique to members of the group.

Most paratyphoid salmonellae from poultry belong to subgroups B, C or D serogroups. The 'H' antigens are determined by flagellar proteins and are identified by lower case letters. Flagellar antigens sometimes occur in 2 different phases. The serotype of a particular salmonella isolate is determined by combination of O (somatic) and H (flagellar) antigens expressed by them. Serotyping of isolates is generally accomplished using agglutination tests with batteries of specific antisera. Slide agglutination tests are first used to establish the somatic antigen and the flagellar antigen is then determined using tube agglutination tests.

Resistance to Physical and Chemical Reagents

Salmonellae are generally destroyed by heat (cooking to 79^0C). Cooking eggs at 60^0C for 3.5 minus (Pasteurisation) can kill salmonellae in eggs. Steam pelleting (conditioning) of feed can make the feed free of salmonella infection. Phenols and quaternary ammonium compound used for sanitization of poultry houses reduce though not totally destroy salmonella infection. Use of lactic acid, acetic acid, hydrogen peroxide, chlorine have been reported to reduce salmonellae load on the carcasses of broilers. Formaldehyde fumigation or hydrogen peroxide or spraying of poly-hexamethylene biguanide hydrochloride is effective in controlling salmonella on hatching eggs.

Chemical treatment of poultry feeds using organic acid mixture significantly reduce salmonella contamination caused by rodent faecal pellets.

Pathogenesis of PT Salmonella Infections

Lipopolysaccharide endotoxins of PT salmonellae are responsible for fever, liver and spleen lesions in 2 weeks old chickens and those Lipopolysaccaride also resist hosts phagocytic activity of immunological system. Enterotoxin reduce secretary response of enterocytes of host and that results in accumulation of fluids in intestine of the host.

The 'Adherence' of PT salmonellae is pivotal first step of 'Invasiveness' of these organisms. Type 1 fimbriae (pilli) of PT salmonellae are responsible for adherence. Salmonellae grown anaerobically are more adherent and more invasive than those grown aerobically. Rapidly growing salmonellae typhimurium are shown to kill mice faster than slow growing salmonellae.

Plasmids (Extra chromosomal DNA elements of bacteria) of salmonella are directly associated with pathogenicity and virulence. Strains of *S. typhimurium* and *S. enteritidis* cured of their 'Virulence associated' plasmids are found to be less lethal to mice. The plasmid associated virulence among *S. typhimurium* and *S. enteritidis* has been shown to be responsible for their invasion in mesenteric lymph-nodes, liver and spleen in mice. Pathogenecity differences have been noted between the various phage types of *S. enteritidis* with 'phage type 4' often associated with a particularly high level of invasiveness and lethality for newly hatched chicks.

Clinical signs of Paratyphoid Infections

The contamination of eggs with PT infection leads to high levels of embryo mortality in incubator and rapid deaths in newly hatched chicks. The disease is observed up to not more than 2-3 weeks after hatch. The signs of the PT disease are similar to pullorum disease.

Gross Lesions and Histopathology

This is similar to the lesions and HP described under S. pullorum gallinarum.

Isolation and Identification of PT Salmonellae

As PT salmonellae do not often show any lesions and symptoms, it is a best policy to use many organs from the carcass or sacrificed bird including liver, spleen, bunch of ovarian follicles and intestine as well as faecal samples for isolation attempts.

Many selective and enrichment media are tried for salmonellae isolation. First, non-selective pre-enrichment is used to encourage the growth of very small number of salmonellae in case of tissues and egg yolk samples in which no much contaminants are present and only few salmonellae may be present. But for testing of intestinal samples/ faecal material, litter samples, etc. where much contamination is expected only selective media should be used for primary culturing for suppression of competing organisms and selective enrichment to be used for additional expansion of salmonella population. After primary pre-enrichment and secondary enrichment, culturing, lastly plating on selective agar media is used to obtain isolated colonies.

Egg shells are sampled by immersion in selective broth media. Entire egg content are incubated after shell disinfection for expansion of few salmonellae present in them and then, the direct culturing of incubated liquid in eggs is cultured on plates.

Suggested pre-enrichment media include buffered peptone water and trypticase soya broth. Selective enrichment broths include tetrathionate (TT) broth, selenite-cystein (SC), broth, the former is better for this work. Among the commonly used plating media for PT are brilliant green agar, XLD agar, XLT_4 agar, bismuth sulphate agar or Macckonkey agar.

Confirmation of Genus and Serotype

Combined use of triple sugar iron agar and lysine iron agar provides an effective presumptive test for identifying of PT salmonellae. Then sugar fermentation pattern of each isolate for a set of six particular sugars/carbohydrates as described by Cox and Williams (1976) will give additional differentiation. The sero-group can be determined by slide agglutination tests with polyvalent antisera to groups of somatic O antigens (B, C or D groups) and the serotype can then be determined by slide agglutination test with monovalent antisera to specific O antigens and tube agglutination tests with antisera to flagallar H antigens.

New techniques for rapid salmonella detection using DNA probes and specific antibodies to salmonella antigens by ELISA methods using polyclonal antibodies to salmonella Lipopolysaccharides (LPS) or flagella have been reported but are not detailed out here for want of space.

Prevention and Control of PT Infections

Effective preventive and control programmes must involve co-ordinated and simultaneous attacks on the problem from several directions due to the diversity of sources of PT salmonella infections. They can be summarized as follows:

1. Eggs and chicks to be produced only from certified salmonella free flocks.
2. Proper disinfection of shell surface of hatching eggs and hatching in pre-disinfected/fumigated incubators.
3. Thorough cleaning and disinfection of the poultry house and brooding sheds thoroughly using standard prescribed procedures between the flocks.
4. Rodent and insect/pest control, as prescribed.
5. Restricted entry of visitors and workers after following proper disinfection procedures.
6. Feed containing no animal protein and pelleting of feed using proper 'steam conditioning' (90°C for few seconds) procedure should be used.
7. Treatments, such as medication, competitive exclusion cultures usages orally (drinking water) or by spray beginning from day 0.
8. Preventive vaccination against at least S. enteritidis and S. typhimurium along with S. gallinarum for restricted shedding of salmonellae.
9. Monitoring of entire poultry environment for salmonella by proper tests.

Drinking water medication with gentamycin or quinolone antibiotics have limited value in salmonella shedding restriction due to relapses after withdrawal of treatment is experienced. Moreover, development of drug fast condition is also observed.

Competitive exclusion of salmonellae by colonization of probiotic microflora is also one of the effective tools for elimination of salmonella infections. Competitive exclusion (CE) treatments involve administering defined or undefined bacterial cultures to poultry in order to diminish intestinal colonization by salmonellae.

Undefined intestinal flora from birds free from salmonella infection or used litter from SPF birds flocks can be a good source for CE microflora for CE treatment. A defined mixture of microflora from intestines is likely to produce a given level of protection against salmonellae.

Vaccination

Both killed and live vaccines have been associated with protection against PT salmonellae, although neither type of vaccine has consistently shown to provide an impenetrable barrier against infection. Hence, vaccination is most effectively used in conjunction with management practices including competitive exclusion practice to reduce opportunities for flocks to be exposed to PT salmonellae.

In recent years, interest in use of killed polyvalent vaccines (bacterins) in poultry has been renewed due to escalating concerns about S. enteritidis. Subcutaneous administration of oil adjuvanted emulsion bacterins to laying hens has been reported to reduce significantly the incidence of faecal shedding and the frequency of isolation of S. enteritidis from various internal tissues and the incidence of production of eggs with the contaminated contents following subsequent oral challenge (Gast, *et al.*, 1992). Chickens vaccinated with bacterins have been reported to exhibit reduction in mortality, lesions, clinical signs and organ invasion for upto 12 weeks post vaccination when challenged with S. enteritidis by intravenous or intra muscular routes (Timms, *et al.*, 1990).

Oral or intramuscular administration of aro A-mutant of salmonella enteritidis and Acya Acrp S. typhimurium (a double mutant with deletion of both adenylate cyclase and the cyclic AMP receptor protein) provided very strong protection against intestinal colonization and oral invasion in case of S. enteritidis and S. gallinarum respectively (Cooper, *et al.*, 1990 and Hassan, *et al.*, 1994 respectively).

Scenario of salmonella infections and their control in India

Salmonella infections were unknown in India during the back yard poultry keeping Era upto late fifties. After the appearance of commercial poultry farming in India, in early sixties, salmonellosis was not found much. However, during mid sixties, sporadic salmonellosis incidences were recorded by the author in Bombay-Pune poultry belt (eg: at Regional Poultry breeding Farm at Aarey Milk Colony, Kirloskar Poultry Farm Aundh, Kwality Poultry Farm Aundh and Arbor Acres Poultry breeding farm, Talegaon), when he was working with disease investigation section of Animal Husbandry Department of Maharashtra State (Aundh), Pune.

Govt. of Maharashtra declared poultry salmonellosis as 'Scheduled disease' by law and formulated salmonella testing programme and a scheme for testing for Salmonellosis and certification of 'Salmonella free' status for each breeding and bigger commercial poultry establishment was made compulsory after 1965-66. A research scheme for salmonellosis was launched at disease investigation section of Maharashtra state at Aundh, Pune under ICAR funding.

The salmonella antigen standardization techniques followed by antigen producers were not uniform and were far from perfection which resulted into unresolved problem of 'Non-specific' reactors. This provided the chance for releasing of 'doubtful reactors' as negative reactors, thus escaping from disposal of actual borderline positive reactors. Malpractices like treatments of flocks or even positive reactors during the next testing also helped in failure of salmonella testing programme and perpetuation of infection on the farms. All the above points lead to the failure of salmonella control programme and rise in salmonellosis incidence by the beginning of 21st century.

The author during his disease investigation work connected to the vaccine failures as in the field, came across incidences of salmonellosis in commercial poultry in almost every poultry belt in India for the period from 1992 to 2007. The author noted significant mortality and morbidity in newly hatched chicks (both layer and broiler type) ranging from 1% to even upto 50 to 60% quite often, showing presence of unabsorbed yolk sacs, pesty vents and dropping of wings/ ruffled feathers and could isolate salmonella organisms from large number of so-called incidences of *E. coli*. Isolations of *S. pullorum – gallinarum, S. dublin, S. typhimurium* and *S. enteritidis* in addition to many more types of salmonellae were isolated by PDRC scientists from the material from affected chicks collected by the author. Some of these isolates were confirmed and typed by Kasauli and IVRI reference salmonella laboratories, when sent to them by PDRC.

The author also came across the salmonellosis incidences from adult layer birds from broiler and layer breeding stocks and isolated *S. gallinarum pullorum, S. enteritidis* and *S. typhimurium* with the help of PDRC scientists from such incidences during the period from 1992 to 2007.

During our investigation work, when it was found that the salmonella problem in Indian poultry industry has gone out of control due to the sad failure of testing and eradication policy and this policy no longer remained practically feasible on the grounds of Breeder's economic problems, it was thought that it will now be a wise policy to adopt control of salmonellosis by a 'Combined testing-vaccination management approach'.

Ventri Biological was the first to get a nod from Ministry of Agriculture, Govt. of India and FDA (Drug Controller of India) to produce a combined polyvalent salmonella inactivated vaccine comprising of *S. gallinarum, S. enteritidis* and *S. typhimurium* adjuvanted with mineral oil and emulsifiers Tween 80 and Arlacel 80. The idea is to control shedding of salmonellae by vaccination after initial testing of breeding flocks and adapt managemental practices of preventing dissemination of broiler salmonellae from feed by use of pelleted 'steam conditioned' feed and other usual bio-security measures including rat proofing, pest/insect control and restricted visitor/ workers movement. All these when combined may be able to reduce the incidences of salmonellosis though eradication of salmonella presently seems to be unimaginable.

During 2009,Polchem, India introduced bacteriophage of salmonella pullorum-gallinarum (product 'Biotector' of C.J. Corporation of south Koria) for therapeutic use by drinking water route and through feed in poultry. S.V. Pandit and S.B. Salutgi, *et al.* of Biospace Lab, Pune followed the sout and introduced cocktail of multiple bacteriophages of number of salmonella field isolates for the use in drinking water and poultry feed successfully during the same year. It is noticed that bacteriophage treatment positively reduces salmonella shading and symptoms and lesions of salmonellosis in poultry. And it is hoped that it may be usefull for control of the same in near future.

Pandit and Salutgi, *et al.* (2009) prepared formalin inactivated multivalent Salmonella vaccine using more than twenty five field salmonella isolates (oil adjuvanted) which afforded better field coverage. This multipronged attack on the salmonellosis problem will be usefull for future of poultry in India.

During 2017, Pandit and Salutgi attempted isolation of *Bdellovibro bacteriovorax*, an organism from poultry farm suage which is predatory on most of the gramme negative bacteria including salmonella and *E. coli*. Lot of work conducted abroad including in China has raised a hope of finding a solution for salmonellosis control in near future by using bdellovibrio bacteriovorax (personnal communication-2017).

Suggested Reading

Christensen, J.P., Olsen, J.E., Hansen, H.C. & Bisgaard, M. (1992). Characterization of Salmonella enterica serovar gallinarum biovars gallinarum and pullorum by plasmid profiling and biochemical analysis. Avian Pathol., 21: 461-470.

Gupta, B.R. & Mallick, B.B. (1976). Immunization against fowl typhoid. 1: Live oral vaccine. Indian J. anim. Sci., 46: 502-505.

Gupta, B.R. & Mallick, B.B. (1976). Immunization against fowl typhoid. 2: Live adjuvant vaccine. Indian J. anim. Sci., 46: 546-551.

Gupta, B.R. & Mallick, B.B. (1977). Use of 9R strain of S. gallinarum as vaccine against S. pullorum infection in chicks. Indian vet. J., 54: 331-333.

Rettger, L.F. (1900). Septicaemia among young chickens. N.Y. Med. J., 71: 803-805.

Tsubokura, M. (1965). Studies of Salmonella pullorum phage. I: Isolation of phages and their properties. Jpn. J. vet. Sci, 27: 179-188.

Tsubokura, M. (1966). Studies on Salmonella pullorum phage. V. Conversion of subtypes of S. pullorum by phage. Jpn. J. vet. Sci., 28: 35-40.

❑❑❑

Chapter 17

Chronic Respiratory Disease: Mycoplasm Gallisepticum Infection (Air sacculitis) Complicated with Colibacillosis

Chronic respiratory disease of chickens and infectious sinusitis of Turkeys is caused by *Mycoplasma gallisepticum* (MG) and is characterized by respiratory rales coughing, Nasal discharge in chickens and sinusitis in turkeys. Clinical manifestation develops usually slowly and the disease has a long course. Generally the disease is secondarily complicated with *Escherichia coli* (Collbacillosis) and sometimes with other respiratory virus infections and such a complicated air saculitis is also called as ccRD (Complex Chronic Respiratory Disease).

Thus, two infectious agents, one belonging to mycoplasma species and another belonging to *Escherichia coli* species are involved in this complex problem of respiratory disease. Let us know about each of these agents in this chapter as separate entity and then know about their complex conjoint manifestation.

A. Mycoplasmosis

Mycoplasma species were probably first encountered in chickens by Nelson (1933), which he called as 'Fowl Coryza'. However, Delaplane, *et al.* (1934) described the condition designated as chronic respiratory disease. Van Roekel, *et al.* (1951) reported on successful cultivation of the organism from chicken and Turkeys and noted their similarities.

Mycoplasma organisms tend to grow rather slowly, at 37^0-38^0 and are resistant to penicillin and thallium acetate. They are very small 'Prokaryotes' totally devoid of cell walls, bound by a plasma membrane only, which accounts for their 'fried egg' type colonial morphology. The penicillin resistance of the mycoplasma organisms is due to the fact that penicillin acts on microbes and inhibit their growth by affecting their cell walls while mycoplasma do not posses cell walls and hence they are not inhibited by penicillin.

Typical colonies of mycoplasma species are small (0.1-1.0 mm in diameter) smooth, circular and somewhat flat with more dense central elevation which gives the appearance of 'Ambonate colonies'. The organisms are slender rods, filaments and ring forms and are very fainty stained by carbol fuchsin. They are faintly (gram stained negatively) stained. Numbers of non-pathogenic mycoplasma species are isolated from poultry but pathogenic species are only 3, namely: 1) *M. gallisepticum*, 2) *M. synoviae* and 3) *M. meleagridis*, the third species affects only turkeys and hence we will not deal with it. M. synoviae affects mainly turkeys but it can produce synovitis as well as air sacculitis is chickens. *M. gallisepticum* causes chronic respiratory disease in chickens as well as 'Sinusitis' in growing turkeys. All the 3 mycoplasmas in birds can produce haemagglutination of chicken erythrocytes and haemagglutination inhibition tests can specifically differentiate between these 3 species.

About mycoplasma gallisepticum and mycoplasma sinoviae organism

The morphology and colonial characters are as described. *M. gallisepticum* as well as *S. sinoviae* require 10-15% swine serum (heat inactivated) for their growth. However, avian serum or Horse Serum can also be used. Yeast autotysate is useful for growth of M. gallisepticum while NAD is essential for growth of *M. Synoviae*. The medium containing phenol red and dextrose or 0.0025% 2-3-5 triphenyl tetrazine chloride along with swine/horse/avian serum and NAD/Yeast autotysate and Penicillin can be used for primary isolation of the organisms. The change of pH indicated by the above mentioned pH indicators will indicate growth of mycoplasma in the medium. The organisms can be further plated on Nobel agag enriched with swine/horse/avian serum and NAD/yeast autotysate to observe and incubated for 3-5 days at 37^0C for looking for characteristics 'ambonate colonies'.

Bio-chemical properties

Mycoplasma gallisepticum ferment glucose, Maltose with acid but No gas. It does not ferment lactose dulictol or salicin. Sucrose is rarely fermented and reduce 2-3-5 tripheryl tetrazolium (blue to red). It completely haemolyses horse erythrocytes in agar medium and agglutinates chickens erythrocytes.

M. Synoviae does not reduce 2-3-5 triphenyl tetrazolium (does not become red from blue). Rest of the characteristics of Bio-chemical reactions is the same as that of *M. gallisepticum.*

M. gallisepticum and *M. synoviae* can be differentiated by conducting HI tests. HI antibodies are specific for each species. Moreover, *M. Synoviae* can produce 'Synovitis' in poultry which is not possible in case of *M. gallisepticum*. But both the species can be responsible for air sacculitis in poultry.

Pathogenesis and Eipzootology

Direct contact of susceptible birds with infected carrier chickens or turkeys can cause outbreaks of the disease. Spread by contaminated air borne dust, droplets or feather is also possible. Spread by contaminated equivalent by contact is commonly assumed but is not well documented.

Lateral spread *of M. gallisepticum* in small flocks of chickens has 4 phases:

1. A latent phase (10-12 days) before antibody was first detected in inoculated birds
2. A period (1-21 days) in which infection gradually appeared in 5-10% of flock population
3. A period (7-32 days) in which 90-95% birds develop antibodies
4. A terminal phase (3-19 days) in which rest of the population is positive.

The infection can also be transmitted through the eggs in chickens and turkeys. Even transmission through semen from affected males is also demonstrated.

Incubation period of 6 to 21 days is noted for *M. gallisepticum* infection. Many chicken flocks develop clinical infection near the onset of egg production, suggesting a low level of inherent infection (probably due to egg transmission) that precipitates from a series of stressing events.

Clinical Disease

Naturally occurring disease in adult flock reveals tracheal rales, nasal discharge, coughing, reduction in feed consumption and loss of weight. Egg production is declined but is maintained at lowered level.

In number of birds, outbreaks occur between 4th and 8th weeks of age. The feed conversion ratio is increased with high feed consumption and lower weight gains at the time of marketable age of the commercial broilers. In layer chickens, cases of Kerato conjunctivitis occur with swelling of the facial skin and eyelids. The infection is more severe and of longer duration in winter and affects younger birds more severely than the matured birds (in which more loss due to lower egg production in observed).

M. gallisepticum is the primary cause of chronic respiratory disease but other organisms frequently cause complication. Severe air Sac infection, frequently designated as complicated CRD (cCRD) or air sac disease is the more commonly encountered in the field. ND or IB may precipitate the disease outbreak of cCRD. *E. coli* is found to be a frequent complicating organism.

It is known that *E. coli* alone can't infect air sacs unless *M. gallisepticum* previously involves them. In broilers, mortality may be negligible with uncomplicated disease but it can go upto 30%, when complicated with *E. coil*. The *Mycoplasma Synoviae* (MS) produce infectious sinovitis with lameness and retarded growth. Feathers become ruffled, combs shrink and swelling around the hock joints and foots pads can be observed. Air sacculitis with MS infection is also commonly observed similar to MG infection.

Gross lesions and Histopathology

Gross lesions consist of catarrhal exudates in nasal and para nasal passages, trachea, bronchi and air sacs. Sinusitis is more common in turkeys than in chicken. Air sacs contain caseous exudates or beaded or lymphofolicular appearance is observed. Some degree of pnenmonia can be present. Fibrinous or fibrino-purulent perihepatitis and pericarditis can be seen along with air sacculitis. Moderate to severe encephalitis may be present. M.S. infection with synovitis show creamy to gray coloured exudates in synovial membranes of tendon sheaths, joints and keel bone, hepato-spleenomegaly, swelling of kidneys with paleness and mottling is also observed. Caseous exudates in tendon sheaths and joints as the infection become chronic.

Infiltration of mono nuclear cells and hyperplasia of mucous glands, pneumonia and lympho-folicular changes in lungs are common.

Diagnosis : The gross lesions in air sacs, perihepatitis and pericarditis are clinically diagnositic. However, for confirmation, cultural examination by isolation of mycoplasma from excudate swabs and culturing of affected liver and pericardium using special mycoplasma broth and solid media described in earlier paragraphs may be undertaken. 'HAI test' on paired sera samples may be used for sero-diagnosis.

The egg transmission (Vertical transmission) being the major mode of the spread of infection and affected birds becoming 'Carriers' of the disease when matured, detection of 'Carriers' by serological testing has become the necessity. Serum plate agglutination (SPA) test using coloured MG and MS antigens is used for detection of carriers of these 2 infections. However, problem of 'non-specific' reactors interfere with the detection of true 'Carriers'. It is demonstrated that use of oil adjuvanted bacterins prior to testing of serum for bird with coloured plate agglutination may give false positive reaction (Cullen, *et al.*, 1972).

HI test has been commonly used to confirm 'reactors' detected by SPA test. However, it is time consuming and antigen is not commercially available for HI test. ELISA test kits are now available for replacement of HI and SPA tests (Czifra, *et al.*, 1993), using monoclonal antibody for detection of MG antigen.

Chemotherapy : *M. gallisepticum* and *M. Sinoviae* are susceptible to several antibiotics including streptomycin, oxytetracyclin, erythromycin, spiramycin, tylosin, tiamutine, tiamulin and lincomycin. Resistant strains for some of these antibiotics are also described. Use of these antibiotics in feed for reduction of egg transmission of hatching eggs is found effective. Tylosin (subcut injection of 2-3 mg/lb of body weight or 2-3 grammas/gallon of drinking water for 3-5 days has given good results in treatment of CRD. Egg transmission of *M. gallisepticum* is reduced by low grade addition of some of these antibiotics in feed but not completely eliminated the shedding of mycoplasma organisms.

Egg dipping with tylosin sulphate containing water has been used as a means of getting rid of mycoplasma contamination through surface of eggs before setting of eggs for hatching.

Immunization

Use of inactivated *M. gallisepticum* and *M. Synoviae* oil adjuvanted bacterins in late 1970s was tried on multiple age group containing farms, which could reduce the incidences of Mycoplasma induced 'egg drops' in layer birds and the air sacculitis problem in their commercial progeny. It was also found that reduction in 'air sacculitis' in broiler is possible using such bacterins.

Use of live *M. gallisepticum* vaccines is also reported with variable success. 'R' strain and F strain vaccines are described. But these live vaccines are not commercially successful.

Colibacillosis

Colibacillosis is 'localized or systemic infection' caused entirely or partly by *Escherchia coli* which includes Coli-septicaemia, Coli granuloma (Hjarres disease), air cellulitis (inflammatory process of subcutis), swollen head syndrome, perotonitis, salpingitis, osteomyelitis, synovitis, pan-opthalmitis and omphalitis/yolk sac infection.

Early records of *E. coli* infection detected in 70% chicks with 'Mushy chick disease' characterized by oedema and yolk sac affection found in literature is by Harry (1957) who isolated pathogenic *E. coli* from yolk sacs of affected chicks. Gross (1961) described development of Air sacculitis caused by *E. coli*, after the damage of respiratory tract by concurrent infections. Fross (1966) demonstrated that pericarditis and myocarditis is caused by most of the pathogenic *E. coli* serotypes. Morley and Thompson (1984) described occurrence of swollen Head syndrome in broiler chickens in South Africa associated with *E. coli* and an unidentified 'Corona virus' infection.

About Etiology of Coli-bacillosis

E. coli is a gram negative, non acid fast, non-spore bearing, uniformly staining motile organism. It grows on ordinary nutrient media at 37^{0}C and is aerobic and facultative anaerobic. It produces acid and gas when grown in glucose, maltose, manitol, xylose, sorbitol and arabinose but does not ferment dextrin, starch and inositol. It ferments lactose which differentiates it from salmonella species.

Antigenic structure

E. coli are serotyped according to 'Ewing Scheme' which takes into account somatic 'O' antigens, capsular 'K' antigens, Flaggelar

'H' antigens and Pilus 'F' antigens. As per Lion (1994) Wray *et al.* (1996) 173 'O', 74 'K', 53 H and 17 F antigens are recognized and are used for determination of serotypes.

Antigen O is an 'endotoxin' derived from lysis of the organism and is a complex of poly saccharide phospholipid with a protein fraction when antigen 'O' is incubated at 50^{0}C for 24 hours with specific antiserum, it agglutinates at very high titre (over 1:2560) (Ewing, 1956; Sojka, 1965; Wray, *et al.*, 1996).

Antigen 'K' is on the surface of E. coli organism and covers 'O' antigen. It can be removed by heating at 1 hour at 100^{0}C. Antisera against 'K' antigen can be produced by inoculation of 'Whole' organisms in rabbits intravenously. Tube agglutination titres can be determined by including antigen antibody mixtures at 37^{0}C for 2 hours or at 4^{0}C for overnight (Titres 1:100-1:400 usually). These 'K' antigens can be identified by slide agglutination test using diluted serum (Wray, *et al.*, 1996). 'H' antigens of E. coli are proteins which are destroyed at 100^{0}C. Tube agglutination test is read after incubation at 37^{0}C for 2 hours, these antigens are not co-related with pathogenicity. 'F' pillar antigens are involved in adherence/colonization.

Serotypes and their relation with Pathogenecity

Surveys in various parts of the world have shown that most common serotypes associated with pathogenicity in chickens are 0.1, 0.2, 0.35 and 0.78 (Heller, *et al.*, 1977; Wray, *et al.*, 1996). A total of 74 of 154 *E. coli* serotypes caused pericarditis and mortality in 3 weeks old chicks following inoculation of air sacs and/or death of 13 days old embryos following allantoic inoculation (Siccardi, 1966). K-1 & K-80 capsular antigens appear to have correlation with virulence in most of the strains (Wooley, *et al.*, 2000). Omphalitis and Yolk Sac infections in day old chicks, transmitted from their breeder mothers were associated with serotypes 078 and 0139 avian pathogenic *E. coli* (APEC) (Giovamaridio, 2005).

Bacterial Virulence Factors

Following factors were found Associated with virulence of *E. coli* from Poultry:

1. Serotypes 01, 02, 035, 078 and 0139 (Heller and Drabkin, 1977).
2. Capsular Antigens K1 and K-80 (Woodey *et al.*, 1992).

3. Adonitol Fermentation (Rosenburger *et al.,* 1985)/Sorbitol fermentation (Enterotoxigenic strains).
4. Antibiotic resistance (Chulasiri and Suthienkul, 1989).
5. Congo red dye up take (related invasiveness) (Berkhoff and Vinal, 1986).
6. Presence of large Plasmids (Wooley, *et al.,* 1992).
7. Presence of Pili (Colonization in trachea) (Dho, *et al.,* 1982)
8. Smooth lipo polysaccharide endotoxin (Wooley, *et al.,* 1993).
9. Avian cell adherence (Yerushalmi *et al.,* 1990).
10. Resistance to phagocytosis or killing (Arp L.H. *et al.,* 1981).
11. Cytotoxin (Enterotoxin) - Akashi N. *et al.,* 1993.

It is interesting to note that no single virulence factor is associated with all pathogenic *E. coli.*

In addition to virulence factors of bacteria (*E. coli*) following factors of Host are incriminated to alter the host susceptibility to *E. coli* infections in poultry:

1. Viruses such as Adenoviruses, CAA, Hemorrhagic enteritis virus, IBV, ILT, Avian influenza, NDV, Reo virus and Turkey rhino-sinusitis virus (pneumovirus), increase susceptibility of hosts for *E. coli.*
2. Bacteria like bordetella avium, clostridium gallisepticum, mycoplasma sinoviae also increase susceptibility of infected birds to *E. coli.*
3. Parasites including coccidial species, Ascaridia galli (larve), Histomonus meleagridis.
4. Ammonia, cyclophosphamide, Iron parenterals of mycotoxins increase susceptibility of birds to *E. coli.*
5. Contaminated water, dry dusty conditions, feed/water restriction, inadequate ventilation, overcrowding, poor litter conditions, and temperature extremes create the increased susceptibility of chickens to *E. coli* infections.
6. Low protein feed, stress and age are the physiological enhancers of susceptibility of birds to *E. coli.*

Role of *E. coli* infection in various forms of coli bacillosis in poultry

1. Embryo and early chick mortality

Faecal contamination of egg shell surface is the most important source of *E. coli* associated embryonic mortality. Other sources may be ovarian infection (salipingitis). The incidence of infection of yolk sac of embryos increases shortly after hatching and is reduced after about a week post hatch. Many embryos may die before hatching and some die at hatching. The yolk sac infection or omphalitis losses may continue upto 3 weeks of age of chicks.

Microscopically the wall of infected yolk sac is edematous, there may be outer connective tissue zone followed by a layer of inflammatory cells containing heterophils and macrophages, a layer of giant cells, a zone of necrotic heterophils and masses of bacteria and then inner infected yolk. Few plasma cells may also be present.

2. Respiratory Tract Infection

Concurrent infection of *E. coli* with various combinations of infectious bronchitis (IB) virus, combinations of infectious bronchitis (IB) virus, New castle disease (ND) virus including ND vaccine strains and mycoplasma creates Respiratory Disease Complex (RDC) which becomes a chronic infection and is known as Chronic Respiratory Disease (CRD) which also produces Air sacculitis, pneumonia, pericarditis and perihepetitis which is of common occurrence on poultry farms. Less commonly, pan-opthalmitis infections of bones and synovial structures following septicaemia, chiefly in 4 to 9 weeks old chickens with considerable loss, high morbidity, mortality and heavy economic losses due to loss of weight gains and increased Feed Conversion Ratio (FCR).

Gross lesions and histopathological picture

Infected air sacs are thickened, become opaque and often have caseous exudates on respiratory surface microscopically. The earliest changes consist of oedema and heterophilic infiltration, mono-nuclear phagocytes and later on accumulation of giant cells along the margin of necrotic areas. There is proliferation of fibroblasts and necrotic heterophils in the caseous exudates. Lesions of predisposing respiratory disease consist of lymphoid follicles, epithelial hyperplasia and epithelium lined air passages, containing heterophils.

Pericarditis, associated with myocarditis with cloudy pericardial sac, oedematous epicardium which gets covered with light coloured exudates. Saliphigitis is observed (when left abdominal air sac is infected) with a large caseous mass in a dilated, thin walled oviduct.

Yolk may break out from infected ova and 'egg peritonitis' may develop. Acute sepiticaemia can occur which may resemble fowl typhoid / fowl cholera but *E. coli* will be isolated from the lesion. Green liver, marked spleno-megaly may be observed. Sometimes, synovitis and osteomyelitis with joint infections can develop. Pan opthalmitis is an uncommon sequel of *E. coli* septicaemia, which is characterized by blindness hypo-pyon of one eye usually.

Granulomas in liver, cacca, duodenum and mesentery may be observed in a condition known as coli-granuloma (Hjarr's Disease). Swollen Head Syndrome (SHS) with subacute cellulitis involving periorbital and adjacent subcutaneous tissues as of head can also develop after IBV or pneumovirus predisposition. Enterotoxigenic *E. coli* may produce enteritis lesions with diarrhoea.

Diagnosis

Isolation and identification of *E. coli* from lesions of coli-bacillosis desctibed above using culturing and serotyping method described previously in this chapter will lead to proper diagnosis.

Treatments

Nitrofurans, gentamicin, ampicillin, chloramphenicol, chlorotetracycline, neomycin, oxytetracyclin enrofloxin (enrosum) are the antibiotics/ anti bacterials of choice. But development of drug resistance is quite common due to over usage of the antibiotics and even sulpha drugs.

Vaccines and Preventive Measures

Effective inactivated vaccines against serotypes 02:K1 and 078:K80 have been reported to be working well. Multivalent vaccine made from pili containing low levels (180 micro grammes) of protein per dose reduced the severity of challenge infection. Pili of serotypes 01, 02, and 078 are antigenically different. Number of attempts to produce both live as well as inactivated vaccines effective against *E. coli* infections are reported but are not found to be under large scale use in the field, probably due to the multiplicity of pathogenic serotypes and strains under such serotypes.

There are no known methods for reducing the level of pathogenic *E. coli* in the intestinal tract and faeces. However, consideration: 1) Pelleted feed has fewer *E. coli* than mash, 2) Rodent droppings are a source of pathogenic *E. coli* and 3) Contaminated water can contain high numbers of pathogenic *E. coli*, should not be overlooked. Hence, 1) use of Pelleted feed 2) use of 'Probiotic microflora' from *E. coli* resistant chickens 3) water sanitization usage are means to reduce the incidence of *E. coli* infection, including all Bio-security measures described under chapter in 'Salmonellosis'.

Indian Scenario on CRD and Colibacillosis

Chronic respiratory disease is prevailing in commercial poultry since the beginning of poultry industry in India, i.e. since late fifties and early sixties of nineteenth century. The mycoplasma infection exists almost ubiquitous in bird's generation after generation. However, it lies in dormant form in air sacs of the birds and gets precipitated, when ever any stress occurs in respiratory tract of the bird, such as hot IBD vaccination or Lasota vaccination by fine spray method, dustiness in poultry shed environment (dry powdery feed), etc. and generally it gets complicated with *E. coli* infection which is also ubiquitous, coming from unhygienic water source or dust in litter, etc.

Investigation of early chick mortality indicates that during winter season, huddling of chicks occurs during chilly nights if brooding management is not with uniform heating in chick guards, suffocation of chicks occur with heavy mortality. If *E. coli* and mycoplasma infection is prevailing in chick shed or in drinking water, secondary complication of CRD and coli-bacilloris occurs.

There is no specific vaccine available for coli bacillosis in India and preventive treatment of 3 days (day one to day three of chick's life) and on 21st to 23rd day with gentamycin and/or higher antibiotics including quinolone derivatives is used along with water sanitizer treatment (povidone iodine/idophore, water acidifiers or chlorine derivatives and Gluteraldehyde, etc.). The vaccines produced against mycoplasma could not become commercially successful in India up till now and chemotherapy is the only solution available today.

Chronic respiratory disease problem was on rise significantly during post vvIBD wave period (1992 to 1999) due to severe immune suppression caused by vvIBD field virus as well as Hot IBD vaccine usage. This problem is further aggravated by immune suppressive emerging disease conditions like IBH/HPS infections, Reo and CAA and hence, the disease could be described as cCRD.

Presently, cCRD is number one disease problem in poultry creating highest economic loss due to severely affected meat production broilers and egg production in layers respectively during the period from 1992 to 2016 up-to-date.

Even though it is reported from broiler and layer flocks by the poultry farmers, CCRD is not given much attention by the private hatcheries as well as Govt. agencies adequately. There is a need for intensive research on serotyping and production of inactivated oil adjuvanted bacterins containing most frequently occurring indigenous serotypes to control the incidence of *E. coli* and mycoplasma infections in India.

Pandit and Salutgi *et al.* isolated at least fifty phages against *E.coli* isolates from the field from infected birds and used a cocktail of these phages by oral route therapeutically for control of *E. coli* infections in poultry successfully (Personal communication-2017). They also isolated Bdellovibrio bacteriovorax species of mico-organisms from poultry suvage which have predatory action on gram negative organisms including *E.coli*. Cocktail containing Bdellovibrio and *E. coli* phages can be the future therapeutic answer for *E. coli* infections in poultry, if administered orally and by intranasal route.

Suggested Reading

Berkhoff, H.A. and Vinal, A.C. (1986). Congo red medium to distinguish between invasive and non-invasive Escherichia coli pathogenic for poultry. Avian Dis., 30(1): 117-121.

Chulasiri, M. and Suthienkul, O. (1989). Antimicrobial resistance of Escherichia coli isolated from chickens. Vet. Microbiol., 21: 189-1941.

Czifra G., Sundquist B., Tuboly T. & Stipkovits L. (1993). Evaluation of a monoclonal blocking enzyme-linked immunosorbent assay for the detection of Mycoplasma gallisepticum-specific antibodies. Avian Dis., 37: 680–688.

Delaolane, J.P., Erwin L.E. & Stuart, H.O. (1934). A hemophilic bacillus as the cause of an infectious rhinitis. Rhode Island State College Bulletin no. 244: 1-12.

Dho, M.; Lafont, J.P. (1982). Escherichia coli colonization of the trachea in poultry: comparasion of virulent and virulent strains in gnotoxenic chickens. Avian Dis., 26: 787-797.

Gross, W.B., and Siegel, P.B. (1959). Coliform peritonitis of chickens. Avian Dis. 3: 370-373.

Harry, E.G. (1957). The effect of embryonic and chick mortality of yolk contamination with bacteria from the hen. Vet. Rec. 69: 1433-1439.

Heller, E.D. and Drabkin, N. (1977). Some characteristics of pathogenic *E. coli* strains. Br. Vet. J. 133(6): 572-578.

Morley, A.J., and Thomson, D.K. (1984). Swollen head syndrome in broiler chickens. Avian Dis. 28: 238–243.

Nelson, J.B. (1933). Studies on an uncomplicated coryza of the domestic fowl. I. Isolation of a bacillus which produces a nasal discharge. Journal of Experimental Medicine 58: 289-295.

Rosenberger, J.K., Fries, P.A., Cloud, S.S. and Wilson, R.A. (1985). *In vitro* and *in vivo* characterization of avian *Escherichia coli*. II. Factors associated with pathogenicity. Avian Dis. 29(4): 1094-1107.

Sojka, W.J. (1965). *Escherichia coli* in Domestic Animals and Poultry. Commonwealth Agricultural Bureau: Farnham Royal, England.

Van Roekel, H., Clarke, M.K., Bullis, K.L., Olesiuk, O.M. & Sperling, F.G. (1951). Infectious bronchitis. American Journal of Veterinary Research, 12: 140-146.

Wooley, R.E., Spears, K.R., Brown, J., Nolan, L.K. & Fletcher, O.J. (1992). Relationship of complement resistance and selected virulence factors in pathogenic avian *Escherichia coli*. Avian Diseases, 36: 679-684.

Wooley, R.E., Gibbs P.S., Brown T.P., Maurer J.J. (2000). Chicken embryo lethality assay for determining the virulence of avian Escherichia coli isolates. Avian Dis. 44: 318-324.

Wooley, R.E., Nolan, L.K., Brown, J., Gibbs, P.S., Giddings, C.W. and Turner, K.S. (1993). Association of K-1 capsule, smooth lipopolysaccharides, traT gene, and colicin V production with complement resistance and virulence of avian *Escherichia coli*. Avian. Dis. 37: 1092-1096.

Wray, C., Davies R.H., and Corkish J.D. (1996). Enterobacteriaceae. Pp. 9-43 in Poultry Diseases, eds. F.T.W. Jordan and M. Pattison, WB Saunders, Cambridge, UK.

❏❏❏

Chapter 18

Fowl Cholera

Fowl Cholera (FC) is a contagious bacterial disease of poultry, caused by *Pasturella multocida*. It usually appears as a septicaemic disease with high morbidity and mortality, but benign, chronic form of the disease is also not uncommon with local involvement of comb and wattles.

Europe faced several epornitics of this disease in later part of the 18th century with the 1st official record in France by Chabert in 1782. However, Mallet was the first to call it as fowl cholera. Huppe referred to the term Haemorrhagic septicaemia (1886) and Liginieres called it 'Avian Pasturellosis' (1900). Peroncito of Italy and Semmer of Russia observed the bacterium with rounded form occurring singly or in Paris in the tissues affected with this disease in 1877 and 1878 respectively, while Toussaint isolated the bacterium and proved it to be the sole cause of this disease.

Pasteur (1880) isolated organisms by growing them in pure cultures in chicken broth and then used them for his classical experiments in attenuation of bacteria for use in producing the vaccine for immunization of poultry. Salmon studied the disease for the 1st time in USA in 1880, even though the good description of the disease signs is available in USDA report as early as 1867.

Incidence of the Disease

The disease occurs sporadically or enzootically in most of the countries with high mortality sometimes while losses are nominal at other times. Albert's and Graham (1948) reported 68% mortality within 6 days in turkeys while Vaught *et al.* (1967) reported that 1000 wild geese died due to FC in one night. Hall *et al.* (1955) observed low mortality but persistent infection for 4 years on one premises. The disease is more prevalent in late summer, fall and winter. Chickens become more susceptible as they reach the maturity.

About the Causative Organism

Pasturella multocida var Avium the name suggested by Rosenbusch and Merchant is now accepted as the official name in Burgey's manual, as the causative agent of fowl cholera.

P. multocida is a gram negative non-motile, non-spore bearing rod shaped pleomorphic organism occurring singly or in Pairs or occasionally as chains or filaments in repeated subcultures but it is found as 'bipolar' organisms in tissues/blood and in recently isolated cultures. It is shown to bear pili also.

The organism grows aerobically or unaerobically also at 37^{0}C optimally, in pH range of 7.2-7.8. However, it can also grow in pH range of 6.2-9.0, depending upon composition of the medium. In liquid medium, maximum growth is obtained between 16 & 24 hours, but the 16-18 hours growth has optimum presence of good capsule. It grows better with chicken blood or serum but cattle/sheep/goat blood/serum is having inhibitory effect on growth. Peptone, casein hydro lysate and avian serum have enhancing action on the growth which is used for enrichment of the media for growth. 'Dextrose starch agar' is the excellent medium for its optimum growth.

The colonies of the isolate of *P. multocida* from the primary culture are smooth, dew drop like, convex iridescent during 18 to 24 hours growth phase but become larger and viscous later on. Colonies from chronic type of Fowl cholera cases are circular, smooth, slightly converse or flat, transient butyrous, discrete and blue.

P. multocida does not produce gas but produces catalase, peroxidase and characteristic odour.

Colonies on blood agar do not produce haemolysis, they do not grow on Mac Conkey agar. They are indol positive, gelatin negative, urease negative, and ferment glucose/sucrose but do not ferment lactose or maltose.

Serological grouping of the strains

Serological typing is based on methods that detect specific capsular and somatic antigens. Passive Haemagglutination test is used for specific capsular serogrouping. Out of the 5 capsular sero-groups of carter, namely A,B,D,E and F. Fowl cholera producing P. multoceda var avium isolates only belong to A and D sero-groups.

Tube agglutination test is used for somatic serotyping. Agar gel diffusion precipitation test is also used for somatic serotyping. However, somatic serotyping done by tube agglutination test and AGPT may not completely co-relate.

AGPT with sera prepared in chickens and heat stable antigen extracts from formal saline treated bacteria is used for somatic serotyping of P. multocida in USA and other parts of the world due to the simplicity of the test. The heat stable antigens form lines of identify with lipo polysaccharide protein complexes from the culture supernatants (specificity of this test is determined by lipo polysaccharide portion of the antigen).

Huddleston *et al.* (1972) found good, though not absolute, correlation between the AGPT and the immune response in chickens and turkeys. On the basis of cross protection test in vivo. 3 types of P. multocida are found in USA namely type1, 2, 3 and 4 which are used in commercial vaccine production against FC. 16 somatic serotypes have been described which are isolated from the birds with fowl cholera (Brogden *et al.,* 1979).

Pathogenicity

Virulence of *P. multocida* in relation to fowl cholera is complex and variable. The ability of *P. multocida* to invade and multiply in the host is enhanced due to the presence of capsule that surrounds the organisms. Loss of ability of a virulent strain to produce capsule results in loss of virulence. However, large capsule does not mean higher virulence as it is depending upon the presence of certain chemical substance associated with capsule rather than with the physical presence.

The organisms enter the tissues of the birds through upper respiratory tract or pharyngeal mucous membrane or conjunction or in case of chronic disease, through cutaneous wounds. Eustachian tube was also suggested as the portal of entry of the organisms. Turkeys are more susceptible for *P. multocida* infection and adult fowls are more susceptible than grower chickens.

The dried culture of *P. multocida* shows signs of toxicity which simulates the signs of fowl cholera of acute type. The toxin is produced by the organisms *in vivo* during multiplication which produces general hyperemia in chickens died from F.C. (toxin is an endotoxin). This endotoxin is nitrogen containing phospholylated lipopoly saccharide and develops signs of fowl cholera in chickens, when injected. This lipo polysaccharide is related to the serotype of the organism.

Epizootology

Fowl cholera is not a vertically transmitted disease. The healthy nasal carriers of *P. multocida* are the enzoatic focus of FC and survivors of an epornitic of FC may be the reservoirs of infection. Carrier birds among the older flock, held over for a 22 month provide reservoir of infection for young susceptible pullets housed with them. Isolates of *P. mulotocida* from cattle and sheep are not pathogenic to fowl but all pig isolates of the same especially those from the area, where fowl cholera is prevalent are highly pathogenic to fowl.

Contaminated crates, feed bags or poultry equipment used previously for FC affected poultry may serve as a source of infection to the new susceptible flocks and birds died of FC can disseminate the infection in the susceptible flock. Infected rats and cats in the premises of poultry can act as a source of infection. Houseflies and other insects from contaminated poultry house can be the possible spreaders of the disease.

About the disease

The acute or peracute cases of Fowl cholera show sudden deaths without showing any symptoms. Fever, anorexia, ruffled feathers, mucous discharge from mouth and nose, diarrhoea and increased respiratory rales, cyanosis of combs prior to death are some common symptoms observed in the outbreak of fowl cholera. Infection becoming chronic with emaciation and dehydration is not uncommon. Low virulence of the organisms can also produce chronic disease with swollen wattles, combs, foot pads or legs and wing joints. Acute FC lesions are characterized by general hyperemia, especially of that of abdominal viscera including duodenal mucosa. Sub-epicardial haemorrhages and sub-serosal petechial or ecchymotic haemorrhages are characteristic and common.

Livers show swollen appearance with typical multifocal necrotic areas on the surface. Pneumonia is quite common. Flacid mature ovarian follicles are observed in the ovary. Yolk material from ruptured ova may also be evident in visceral cavity and hyperemic ovarian stroma may be evident.

Lesions of chronic FC are characterized by facial oedema and swollen wattles and combs, filled with straw coloured fluid, the smear of which may show typical bipolar pasturella organisms when stained with gram stain or lesishman/giemsa stain with typical hollow of capsule surrounding them on microscopic examination. Caseous exudates may be present in local tissues or in bone marrow.

Diagnosis : The postmortem lesions are clinically diagnostic, which can be confirmed by heart blood/smear examination (after staining with leishman/or Giemsa stain) microscopically, looking for characteristic bipolar stained rods in singles and pairs.

Chemotherapeutic treatment of fowl cholera

Antibacterial chemotherapy has been used extensively in treatment of FC, success depends on promptness of treatment and drug used. Sulphamethazine (0.5-1% in feed or 0.1% in drinking water) can reduce mortality of FC from 60 to 85%. Sulphamethazine, sulphamethazine, sulphadiazine and sulpha quinoline are the other sulpha derivatives used successfully by many workers for treatment of FC.

Penicillin, streptomycin, oxytetracyclin and chloremphenocol as well as Novobiocin and erythromycin are found useful as antibiotic treatment for FC. Sulpha drugs are bacteriostatic in FC treatment and hence relapses can be observed after withdrawal. Antibiotic develop drug resistance in the FC organisms and hence, are giving variable results when used.

Immunization

Vaccinations are carried out only in areas where the infection is prevalent. However, vaccination is not a substitute for good sanitary practice.

Oil adjuvanted formalized bacterins containing subtypes 1, 3 and 4 of P. multocida isolated from chickens are used for protection against general FC infection. The birds are vaccinated first at 8 to 10 weeks of age followed by booster dose given at 12 to 16 weeks of age in order to protect the mature layer or broiler breeder birds.

However, in USA, live attenuated CU strain fowl cholera vaccine is used which can provide protection against all 1 to 4 subtypes of

P. multocida, as live organisms when multiply in vivo, they produce wider serological response against all the 4 sub types. But often there is mortality produced after CU strain live vaccination and hence prior to the use of CU strain live vaccine, one dose of oil adjuvanted bacterin is given 4 weeks before live vaccination.

Indian Scenario of Fowl Cholera

Fowl Cholera was prevailing in few poultry pockets of Kolkata region (including midnapur and costal Andhra (including Nellore) in early eighties.

However, during the late eighties there was a severe flare up of the incidences of fowl cholera in poultry belts surrounding Hyderabad (1988-89). No Fowl cholera vaccine was available in those days in India and hence, the poultry farmers had to depend upon sulpha drugs as feed additive on continuous basis for prevention of mortality due to fowl cholera which started recurring again and again in the affected farms due to absence of bio-security and disinfection measures on the farms. The menace of house flies on these farms was quite rampant which was leading to continuous recycling of the FC infection. Continuous use of sulpha drugs as feed additives also was responsible for development of drug resistance in FC organisms. Moreover, sulpha toxicity in the form of nephritis with haemorrhagic kidneys started becoming usual post mortem lesion in the dying birds. Meanwhile outbreaks of fowl cholera newly erupted in Barwala layer poultry belt in Punjab also. The author (Dr. S.V. Pandit) investigated the out breaks in Hyderabad as well as Barwala and he could isolate P. multocida pure cultures from the same. This lead ventri biological scientists to develop an inactivated oil adjuvanted bacterin using local strains. This vaccine was licensed in 1990.

Dr. F.T.W. Jordan mentioned in his personal talk on poultry diseases that the antigenic epitopes on capsular antigen of pasturella multocida are continuously changing and hence it is a best policy to use autogenous bacterin for better protection against fowl cholera. We have similar experience in India and it seems that bacterin produced from same subtype from one place may not work with the same subtype infection on the farms in other place. In such case autogenous vaccine produced from isolates of the affected farm/area works better.

Dr. Pat Blackall's visit in India, during 1999 and his subsequent visits helped the country to develop subtyping facilities for fowl cholera causative agent *P. multocida var avium* (Type D) and subtypes 1,3 and 4 were isolated locally and were incorporated in vaccine. This problem is now fairly under control.

Fowl cholera investigation in Nellore (Costal Andhra) revealed an interesting finding by the author. The affected farms were typically having flooring with rice husk litter. Being a coastal area, this rice husk litter was excessively moist due to humidity being very high in that zone. Such litter was very much favourable for development of significant infestation of the litter with poultry flees. These flees feed on poultry blood and apparently it seems that those flees act as mechanical carrier of FC infection on those affected farms. There is no specific mention about *P. multocida* being transmitted by flees, in the literature. However, it is known that rat flees are carriers of pasturella pestis from rats to human beings. Whether poultry flees carry *P. multocida* infection or not seems to be an interesting point for further investigation.

Our investigations on Fowl cholera in Barwala poultry belt (Punjab) revealed that there is extreme concentration of poultry population in that belt due to very little distances between farm to farm and the farms are typically one storeyed (one above the other). Once fowl cholera occurs on the farm, there is no proper disposal of carcasses which leads to perpetuation of the infection chronically. Indiscriminate use of sulpha drugs in the feed and continuous use of hot IBD vaccines on the farms since 1993 onwards and arrival of new immune suppressive diseases like CAA and Reo infections, all have lead to the unabated coinciding of fowl cholera in this poultry belt and some other similar belts like Hyderabad and Namkkal. Hence, strict bio-security measures also need attention. Of late, Pandit S.V. and Salutgi S.B. *et al* of Biospace lab, Pune isolated from adult poultry birds, number of gram negative isolates of biplar morphology with haemmrhagic characteristic, when grown on chicken blood agar plates and answering other characteristics of Pasturella haemolytica. These organisms grow on macconky agar plates unlike pasturella multoceda var avium which do not grow on macconky medium. These isolates are similar to galli bacterium species described in Burgy's manual recently. These organisms were responsible for Fowl cholera like disease in poultry in pune belt. Pandit and Salutgi isolated number of phages against them for therapeutic use (personal communication 2015 to 2017).

Suggested Reading

Alberts, J.O. and Graham, R. (1948). Fowl cholera in turkeys. North Am. Vet., 29: 24-26.

Hall, W.J., Heddleston, K.L., Legenhausen, D.H. & Hughes, R.W. (1955). Studies on Pasteurellosis: a new species of Pasteurella encountered in chronic fowl cholera. American Journal of Veterinary Research, 16: 598–604.

Vaugh, H.W., Mc Dougle H.C. Bur-gess H.H. (1967). Fowl cholera in waterfowl at Squaw Creek National Wildlife Refuge, Missouri. The Journal of Wildlife Management 31: 248-253.

Chapter 19

Clostridial Diseases of Poultry

Clostridial diseases found in poultry are: a) Necrotic enteritis b) Ulcerative enteritis, c) Gangrenous dermatitis, and d) Botulism.

Most of the clostroidal species are obligate parasitic bacteria, normally present in intestinal tract of poultry, litter and dust in small numbers. However, they can multiply significantly, when the conditions are favourable for them and produce exotoxins either inside the body of poultry birds (e.g. *Clostridium perfringens*) or outside the body of the poultry birds (e.g. *Clostridium botulinum* type, these organisms produce toxins which are responsible for the disease in poultry. The following is the account of clostridial diseases of poultry:

A. Necrotic Enteritis of poultry

Necrotic enteritis in domesticated birds was first described by Parish in 1961 in the United States, which was caused by *Clostridium welchii* (*Cl. perfrigens*). He demonstrated the experimental reproduction of the disease in laboratory.

About organism

Wijewanta and Seneviratna (1971) showed *Clostridium perfrigens* type A as the causative agent of Necrotic Enteritis (NE) while Parish (1961) demonstrated *Clostridium perfringens* type C was present in outbreaks of necrotic enteritis. Alpha toxin produced by types A and C of clostridium perfrigenes and beta toxin produced by clostridium perfrigens type C are believed to be responsible for intestinal mucosal necrosis of NE (Kohler, 1973).

The organism produces inner zone of complete haemolysis and outer zone of greenish incomplete haemolysis when grown on rabbit or sheep blood agar by anaerobic incubation. Most strains ferment glucose, maltose, lactose and sucrose and do not ferment manitol while salicin fermentation is variable. Growth on egg yolk agar plates demonstrates presence of lecthinase and absence of lipase production.

Pathogenesis and epizootology

Naturally occurring outbreaks of NE in broiler birds are observed in 2 weeks to 5 weeks of age while those in layer birds raised on floor pens are found between 3 to 6 months age groups.

Clostridium perfrigens can be present in few numbers in faeces, soil, dust contaminated feed or intestinal contents. Contaminated feed and litter is incriminated as cause of the disease. Nature of feed such as diets containing barley or wheat instead of soya and maize can precipitate the disease. Factors like high fibrous litter, various strains of *Coccidia,* both damage the intestional mucosa which can allow the *Clostridium perfrigens* organism to flair upto produce toxin, thus precipitating the disease. Feeding contaminated fish with clostridium perfrigens can precipitate the 'fish meal disease'. Immuno-suppressive disease agents like CAA or IBD can also precipitate necrotic enteritis intoxication of fish meal oriented clostridium perfrigens type A and C.

About the disease

Marked to severe depression, reduced appetite, reluctance to move, diarrhoea and ruffled feathers are typical symptoms of the disease which is of very short duration.

Usually, Jejunum and ileum are affected most, rarely caeca also are involved. Intestines become friable and are distended with gas. The mucosa is usually thickened and becomes grey, fibrino-necrotic; enteritis with formation of dipthertic membrane in the intestinal mucosa is characteristics. Microscopically, apices of villi show sloughing of epithelium and colonization of bacilli accompanied with coagulative necrosis surrounded by heterophils. Necrosis may extend into submucosa and muscular layers of the intestine.

Diagnosis

It is based on typical gross and microscopic lesions and isolation of the causative agent. *Clostridium perfrigens* can be readily isolated form intestinal contents, scrapings of velvety intestinal wall lesions or haemorrhagic lymphoid nodules by anaerobic incubation overnight at 37^0C on sheep blood agar plates. Identifcation can be done by observation of typical fermentation sugar reactions described under etiology.

Characteristics gross lesions are multiple areas of necrosis and ulceration in the distal small intestine and areas of necrosis in liver, usually jejunum and illial involvement is characteristic.

Treatment and Prevention

Removal of contaminated fish meal can prevent clostredial infections on poultry farms. Use of probiotics, such as lactobacillus acidophilius and streptococcus faecium can also prevent precipitation of clostridial necrotic enteritis infection. Outbreaks of necrotic enteritis can be effectively treated by administration of lincomycin, bacitracin, penicillin and tylosin.

B. Ulcerative Enteritis

This is an enteric infection of broiler birds caused by *Clostridium colinum*, characteristics gross lesions are multiple areas of necrosis and ulceration in the distal small intestine and cacca and areas of necrosis in the liver. Prevention and treatment is similar to necrotic enteritis.

C. Gangrenous dermatitis

Gangrenous dermatitis (GD) is a bacterial disease of poultry caused by clostridial organisms belonging to the species *C. perfringens, C. septicum and C. novei* etc. and sometimes, *Staphylococcus* either singly or in combination with clostidia characterized by gas forming gangrene, producing determatitis and is generally precipitated by immune suppression caused by viruses like VVIBD, chicken anaemia agent (CAA) or Reovirus infection.

Since 1963, there have been reports of gangrenous dermatitis from various parts of the world including from United States (Frazier, *et al.*, 1964; Saunders, *et al.*, 1965), from United Kingdom (Fowler and Hussaini, 1975), Germany (Hiuz, *et al.*, 1975), India (Char, *et al.*, 1986), Belgium (Froyman, *et al.*, 1982) and Argentina (Bianco, *et al.*, 1985).

Etiology

Causes of G.D. are clostridium septicum (Fowler and Hussaini, 1975), *Clostridium perfringens* type A (Bianco, *et al.*, 1985) and *Staphylococcus aureus* (Boots, *et al.*, 1964).

Staphylococcus aureus can be isolated from dermatitis lesions using blood agar plate and incubating at 37⁰C for overnight aerobically while blood agar plates inculated anaerobically can be used for *C. perfringens* isolation (See section of necrotic enteritis for details of Cultural characteristics).

Cl. speticum is also isolated from this disease cases using blood agar anacrobically and then carrying out differential identification by sugar reactions (fermentation of glucose, maltose, lactose and salicin, but not of sucrose and mannital) hydrolysis of gelatin and indol negative reaction.

Pathogenesis and epizootology

Natural outbreaks occur at 17 days to 20 weeks of age (average age of out break is 4 to 8 weeks old broilers. It can also occur in 6 to 20 weeks old layers.

Clostridia are distributed in soil, faeces, dust, contaminated litter, feed or intestinal contents while staphylococci are inhabitant of skin and mucous membranes of poultry. The disease occurs as a sequel to infectious bursal disease virus (IBD), chicken infectious anaemia (CIAV), reticulo enolotheliosis virus, avian adeno virus infections, (IBH), Blue Wing Disease (BWD) predisposes chicken to GD in sweden Denmark and Norwey.

About Disease

Clinical signs of G.D. include varying degrees of depression, in co-ordination, inappetence, leg weakness and ataxia. Period of illness is less than 24 hours and birds may be found dead acutely. Mortality ranges from 1 to 60%.

Gross lesions consist of dark moist areas of skin, usually devoid of feathers overlying wings, breast, abdomen or legs can be found. Extensive blood tinged oedema with or without gas (emphysema) is present beneath affected skin underlaying musculature which is discoloured or grey or may contain oedema and gas between muscle boundries. Sero sanguineous fluid and emphysema may be present in subcutaneous tissue. Discrete white foci of necrosis may be seen on liver, atrophy of spleen, bursa and thymus may be present.

Diagnosis

Typical clinical picture is diagnostic of G.D. However, isolation of causative clostridial/staphylococcal organisms can confirm the disease. It is also necessary to isolate and confirm the predisposing immune suppresive virus infection factor namely IBD, CAA, Reticuloendotheliosis or IBH virus responsible for precipitation of the disease, in order to control this problem perpetuating in the flock.

Treatment and Prevention of the disease

Use of chlortetracyclin terramysin, erythromycin, penicillin or copper sulphate in drinking water for treating the bacterial part of the disease can be useful. However, proper preventive vaccination against IBD, CIAV and IBH/retriculoendothebios may be warranted for disease prevention. Management procedures to improve litter conditions, reduce moisture and bacterial levels in the environment and litter and minimize trauma are useful adjuncts.

D. Botulism

Botulism is not an infectious disease but it is an intoxication caused by exotoxin of clostridium botulinum, it is also named as 'Limberneck' of poultry. Many early incidences of Botulism occurred in free range poultry and modern methods of poultry management were considered to have effect of reduction on the occurrence of this disease.

About organism

Cl. botulinum is gram positive, spore forming bacterium, produces potent exotoxin under anaerotic environmental conditions, especially in poultry carcasses. The myasis of poultry carcass infested with this organism can contaminate the larvae of myasis producing flies and if such larvae are consumed by the birds, they can intoxicate the birds with botulism. The vegetative cells of organism are motile. Subterminal or occasional terminal endo-spores are present in ageing cultures. The toxin of the organism is released during autolysis of the organism.

Type A, C and E of C. Botulism cause disease in birds. Toxins produced by this organism are C1, C2 and type D toxin.

Type C organisms readily grow in the gastrointestinal tract of poultry and are obligate parasites. Type C spores are commonly found in and around poultry farms.

Symptoms of the disease

In chickens, flaccid paralysis of legs, wings, neck and eyelids are predominant features of the disease. Paralytic signs progress cranially from the legs to include wings, neck and eyelids, 'Limberneck' the original and common name for botulism, precisely describes the paralysis of neck.

Affected chickens have ruffled feathers, which may fall out while handling loose droppings and diarrhea is present with excess urates in loose droppings. Mortality can be variable depending on the dose of toxin consumed by the birds, but may go upto 40%. The affected birds lack visible lesions or any microscopic lesions.

Pathogenesis

The pathogenesis was once exclusively thought to be due to ingestion of preformed toxin from outside. Now there is growing evidence that *Cl. botulinum* type C elaborates toxin *in vivo* also to cause disease in poultry. This phenomenon is described as 'toxico – infection' by Russian researchers (Roberts, *et al.*, 1974).

Diagnosis

Lack of gross and microscopic lesions as well as presence of typical signs of Limberneck in poultry is diagnostic, detection of specific toxin in serum, crop or gastrointestinal tract washings from morbid birds by mice intraneous inoculation and showing its neutralization after treatment with known antiserum by intravenous mice inoculation is diagnostic of *Cl. botulinum* type C toxin. Showing presence of toxin in the affected bird is diagnostic but showing toxin in carcass is not diagnostic.

Treatment

Treatment of affected flock with vitamin A, D-3 and E is reported to be found useful in reducing losses of birds. Antibiotics including bacitracin (100 gm/ton in feed) and streptomycin (1 gm/litre in feed) and streptomycin (1 gm/litre) in water is also reported good response.

Prevention and Control

Prompt disposal of dead birds which is a good source of toxin for intoxication of birds, if carried out works well in control of intoxication.

Removal of contaminated litter and through disinfection using calcium hypochlorite, idophor or formalin disinfectants may help to reduce spores of the organism. Fly control is useful to avoid the ingestion of toxin contaminated flies coming in contact of feeding birds.

Vaccination and active immunization

Active immunization with inactivated bacterin - toxoid have been successfully used in pheasants (Kurazoao, *et al.*, 1985). Similar toxoid can be used in chicken also (Dohms, *et al.*, 1982). However, vaccination of large number of broiler chickens is costly and is not practiced due to the limited incidences occurring in poultry industry.

Clostredial Disease: Indian Scenario

C. perfringens infections including Necrotic enteridis (NE) or gangrenous dermatitis were hardly seen on Indian poultry farms during early nineteen sixties and seventies, probably due to the absence of any immune suppressive disease problem in India during that period. However, after appearance of classical IBD in 1976, in Bombay, - Pune poultry Belt sporadic occurrence of NE was observed by the author during his routine investigation work. After arrival of VVIBD problem in India after 1992, sporadic outbreaks of NE were seen frequently in Andhra Pradesh and Tamil Nadu, especially in Namakkal and Hyderabad poultry belts.

More serious clostredial problem which was often faced by the author in Hyderabad, Vizag, Namakkal, Anaparthi, Mysore and Bengaluru was that of Gangrenous Dermatitis during late nineties and early part of 21st century (2001 to 2007) and this was mainly due to precipitation of this disease after occurrences of VVIBD problems during early and late nineteen sixties and occurrence of CIAV problems during 2001 to 2007.

Kolkata region (24 pargana north and south districts) and Barwala, Karnal gurgaon and Jind poultry belts were also experiencing precipitation of NE and GD after Mareks and CIAV immune-suppressive problems during 1996 to 2006. Author also came across NE problems in Goa during 2002 to 2006.

Author used treatment of NE with Metronidozol human tablets (one 400 mg tablet per 5-8 birds, after dissolving in warm drinking water and giving it to broiler chicks affected with NE for 3 days, then gap of 2 days and again treatment for 2 days. He got very good success with this treatment. Author also came across suspected sporadic incidences of Botulism in poultry in north especially in Karnal and Jind poultry belts coupled with usual antibiotics. Use of Vitamin B1 and B12 elicitted good results in treatment.

Polyvallent clostridial perfrigens formalin inactivated and oil adjuvanted bacterin as autovaccine was used successfully by Pandit, S.V. and Salutgi, S.B. with success (personal communication-2014-15). Author also came across suspected sporadic incidences of Botulism in poultry in north especially in Karnal and Jind poultry belts. Couple with usual antibiotics use of Vit. B1 and B12 elicitted good results in treatment.

Suggested Reading

Char, N.L., Khan, D.I., Rao, M.R., Gopal, V. & Narayana, G. (1986). A rare occurrence of clostridial infection in poultry. Poultry Adviser, 19: 59-62.

Fowler, N.G. & Hussaini, S.N. (1975). Clostridium septicum infection and antibiotic treatment in broiler chickens. Veterinary Record, 96: 14-15.

Frazier, M.N., Parizek, W.J. & Garner, E. (1964). Gangrenous dermatitis of chickens. Avian Diseases, 8: 269-273.

Köhler, B. (1973). Diseases in man and animal caused by Clostridium perfringens and their relations. Zeitschrift fur Die Gesamte Hygiene und Ihre Grenzgebiete, 19: 228-234.

Parish, W.E. (1961). Necrotic enteritis in the fowl (Gallus gallus domesticus) 1. Histopathology of the disease and isolation of a strain of Clostridium welchii. Journal of Comparative Pathology, 71: 377-39.

Saunders, J.R. & Bickford, A.A. (1965). Clostridial infection of growing chickens. Avian Diseases, 9: 317-326.

Wijewanta, E.A. & Seneviratna, P. (1971). Bacteriological studies of fatal Clostridium perfringens type A infection in chickens. Avian Diseases, 15: 654-66.

□□□

Chapter 20

Avian Coccidiosis

Coccidiosis of poultry is a protozoan parasitic disease of global importance caused by unicellular enteric parasites of the genus *Eimeria* creating tissue damage to the intestinal canal resulting into interruption in feeding, digestive process or nutrient absorption, dehydration, blood loss and increased susceptibility to other diseases of the poultry birds.

Like many parasitic diseases, coccidiosis is a disease of young bird's age group as well as in the older birds. The immunity development after exposure is quick and protection is afforded to the exposed birds later against the homologous species of the parasite and disease outbreak produced by it. However, the birds are still susceptible to coccidiosis caused by other species of Eimeria to which they are not yet exposed.

Presence of coccidia is ubiquitous in nature and infestation with few oocyts of coccidia may not have any clinical manifestation of the disease. However, ingestion of large number of oocysts can precipitate the disease symptoms. Even though most of the coccidial infections are mild to moderate on poultry premises, but potential for disastrous outbreaks is so high and financial losses are so great that the poultry farmers prefer to give continuous anticoccidial medications to the birds on commercial establishments.

About the Parasites

Several genera are known to infect birds of avian species but those infect poultry belong to 2 genera, namely, *Eimeria* and *Cryptosporidia*. However, the species of the genus eimeria which are pre-dominant causes the disease coccidiosis of the economic importance is here in reviewed.

Species of coccidia are identified on the basis of: 1) Oocyst morphology, 2) host specificity, 3) immune specificity, 4) appearance and location of gross lesions produced in the natural host and 5) length of the pre-patent period.

Lifecycle : Lifecycle of coccidium starts from coccidial oocyst which has characteristic morphology with central zygote which is wrapped in chitinous double walled shell (which is thin at the micropile, situated at top. The micropile has 'micropile cap' which protrudes out). The oocysts from infected bird are excreted in the faces on the ground and under favourable temperature and moisture they are sporulated to produce 4 sporocysts by division of the zygote. Each sporocyst consists of 2 sporozoites. The sporulated oocyst is, thus in infective stage of the parasite.

The sporulated oocyst with 4 sporocysts, when ingested by the susceptible chick, reaches the proventriculus where the chitinous wall of the oocyst is partially digested by the enzymes of the gastric juice and when this oocyst reaches gizzard, the wall partly weakened by enzymes is crushed due to muscular action of gizzard and the sporocysts are released in the lumen. The chymotrypsin and bile salts in duodenal secretion dissolves the walls of sporocysts and the 'sporozoites' come out of them and enter the epithelial cells or intra-epithelial lymphocytes where the 'sporozoites' undergo asexual development and multiplication (at least 2 generations of asexual cycle occur called as 'Schizogony'. The schizonts of last generation lead to a sexual phase which gets transformed into larger macrogametes (female form) and smaller microgametes (male form). Microgametes are motile and they enter the macrogametes for fusion into a zygote. The zygote matures into a double walled oocyst, which is released into intestinal contents and finally into excreted faeces. The entire process takes 4 to 6 days. During this lifecycle of the parasites, the intestinal epithelium is damaged and brings about exposure of sub mucous surface, resulting into haemorrhages and oozing out of fluid.

Species of Coccidia involved in poultry coccidiosis:

Nine species of the genus Eimeria are involved in poultry coccidiosis, namely: 1) *E. acervulina* 2) *E. brunette* 3) *E. maxima* 4) *E. mitis* 5) *E. mivati* 6) *E. necatrix 7) E. precox* 8) *E. tenella* and 9) *E. hagani*

These species can be differentiated on 5 criteria mentioned earlier as follows:

A. Oocyst morphology

E. maximum has the largest oocyst (size 21.5–42.5 L x 16.5–29.3 w in microns), followed by *E. brunette* (20.7-30.3 L x 18.1 x 24.2 w), *E. tenella* (19.5-26.0L x 16.5-22.8 w), *E. precox* (19.8-24.7 L x 15.7-

19.8w) *E. acervulina* (17.7–20.2L x 13.7 x 16.3 w), *E. mitis* (11.7-18.7 L x 11.0-18w), *E. mivati* (11.1–19.9 L x 10.5 x 16.2w) and *E. hagani* (not known).

B. Appearance and Location of gross lesions

i) ***E.acervulina* :** Duodenal loop is highly affected followed by mild lesion extended upto earlier part of midgut.

ii) ***E. brunetti* :** Distal part of small intestine is mainly affected but milder lesions may spread in caeca and lower part of midgut below yolk sac diverticulum.

iii) **E. maxima :** Midgut is severely affected while it can extend in severe cases upto complete intestine from Duodenum to distal part of lower intestine.

iv) ***E. mitis* :** Mainly distal part of lower intestine is affected. In extreme cases the cacca may get mildly affected.

v) ***E. mivati* :** Duodenal loop and early part of midgut is affected. In severe cases, distal part of midgut may get affected.

vi) ***E. necatrix* :** Complete midgut is severely affected with milder lesions in caeca.

vii) ***E. precox* :** Only duodenum is severely affected with light infection of earlier part of midgut.

viii) ***E. tenella* :** The both caeca are severely affected with light infection of earlier part of lower intestine in very severe cases only.

C. Length of the prepatent period and sporulation time

Sr. No.	Species	Prepatent period (in hours)	Sporulation time (in hours)
1	*E. acervulina*	97 hrs	17 hrs
2	*E. brunette*	120 hrs	18 hrs
3	*E. maxima*	121 hrs	30 hrs
4	*E. mitis*	93 hrs	15 hrs
5	*E. mivati*	93 hrs	12 hrs
6	*E. necatrix*	138 hrs	18 hrs
7	*E. precox*	83 hrs	12 hrs
8	*E. tenella*	115 hrs	18 hrs
9	*E. hagani*	99 hrs	18 hrs

D. Size of schizonts (maximum size)

1.	*E. acervulina*	10.3 micros
2.	*E. brunette*	30.0 microns
3.	*E. maxima*	9.4 microns
4.	*E. mitis*	15.1 microns
5.	*E. mivati*	17.3 microns
6.	*E. necatrix*	65.9 microns
7.	*E. precox*	20.0 microns
8.	*E. tenella*	54.00 microns
9.	*E. hagani*	

E. necatrix has the biggest size of schizonts, followed by *E. tenella*, E.necatrix schizonts are seen in midgut mucosa smears, while *E. tenella* schizonts are found in smears of caecal mucosa.

E. Host specificity and immunological specificity

All the above 9 species of coccidia are found only in poultry and not in any other host. Each of the above 9 species of *Eimeria* are bearing specific immuno genicity *in vivo* and when any bird is exposed to the specific species out of the 9 specific species of *Eimera* mentioned above, and have undergone infection cycle, the bird becomes fully immune to that specific species of *Eimeria* and can not be reinfected again during the rest of the life with that specific species of *Eimeria*. Hence, the pure culture, if used to infect groups of birds repeatedly, then will be immune to that species. Then, if test culture produces patent infections in immunized birds, it must be different species. In this way, by process of elimination, the species can be determined. This technique is time consuming and requires extensive laboratory isolation facility and access to pure cultures of known species of coccidia, but it has proved extremely useful as a research tool and method is used to identify the specific species of poultry eimeria.

About the Disease

Coccidiosis is almost universally found, whereever chickens are grown. The most common means of spread of coccidia is mechanical by personnel who move between pens, houses or farms. However, coccidial infections are self-limiting and severity depends mostly on the number of oocysts ingested and on the immune status of the bird.

Oocysts in litter or droppings of broiler chickens are usually most numerous at 4 to 5 weeks of age. Hence, this is the time when most of the coccidiosis outbreaks takes place. Thereafter, oocyst numbers decline and the birds also become immune and hence, adult breeders and commercial layers show less possibility of coccidiasis outbreaks. But if outbreak occurs during laying period egg drop problem are severe. The ubiquitous nature of poultry coccidia precludes the possibility of elimination or prevention of coccidia by quarantine, disinfection and sanitation.

The coccidiosis is one of the ancientmost diseases of backyard poultry. However, it was Tyzzer who first recorded coccidiosis in North and South America with *E. acervulina*, E. mitis and *E. maxima* species of coccidia, followed by *E. necatrix* and *E. precox* in by Jonhson (1930). Oldest record of coccidiosis in poultry seems to be that of *E.tenella* producing caecal coccidiosis by Railet and Lucet (1891) and Fatham (1909). E. brunette (1942) and E. Hagani (1938) are recorded for the first time by Levine. The recent most species E.mivati is recorded by Edger and siebold in 1964.

Pathogenecity, gross lesions and Histopathology of coccidiosis

The sites of appearance of coccidial lesions of various species of poultry coccidial lesions of various species of poultry coccidia are already mentioned under the sub coloumn. For description of pathogy of coccidia we will prefer 2 species of coccidia representing: 1) intestinal coccidiosis (*E. necatrix*) and 2) Caecal coccidiosis (*E. tenella*) as spectacular lesions are produced by these 2 representative coccidia.

Intestinal coccidiosis (*E. necatrix*)

The major lesion is found in small intestine (similar lesion is also caused by *E. maxima*). Because of the low reproductive capability, *E. necatrix* is not able to compete with other coccidia and is diagnosed mostly in older breeder pullets or layer pullets 9-14 weeks of age.

Intestine is ballooned and lumen may be filled with blood. The oocysts are found only in the caeca. The sexual stages (schizonts) are not seen at the site of intestinal lesions but are found in caeca. Gametocytes are scattered and not found in colonies. Some gross lesions, associated with 1st generation schizogony are seen at 2-3 days post infection (PI) and by 4th day PI, intestine is ballooned and lumen filled with fluid, blood and tissue debris. Foci of infection are seen as white plaques and red petechae from serosal surface.

Microscopic examination of smears from the mucosal surface reveals numerous clusters of large schizonts which are characteristics for this species. Oocysts are never associated with lesions of this species.

Caecal Coccidiosis (*E. tenella*)

E. tenella inhabits the caeca and adjescent intestinal tissues, causing a severe disease characterized by bleeding, high morbidity and mortality, lost weight gain, emaciation. This is the most pathogenic form of coccidiosis in chickens. Bloody droppings are characteristic. Most pathogenic stage is the second generation schizonts which mature at 4 days P.I. like *E. necatrix* and produce colonies of large schizonts which may contain hundreds of merozoites. The schizonts develop deep in lamina propria, so that the mucosa is badly disrupted, when they mature on onset of mortality in flock is rapid and occurs most of it between 5 and 6 days post infection. Severe blood loss brings about severe drop in RBC count and hematocrit value (severe anaemia occurs).

Epizootology

Newly hatched chicks are not susceptible to coccidia due to insufficient chymo-trypsin and bile salt produced by chicks at 1-3 weeks age. However, outbreaks of E. acervulina, *E. tenella* and *E.maxima* occur commonly at 3-6 weeks of age. The birds start becoming immune after this age above 6 weeks which leads to 'self limiting' nature of the disease after this age. There is no cross immunity between the species of eimera and hence, other species can get a chance to produce coccidiosis in these birds above 6 weeks of age (e.g. *E. necatrix* at 8-18 weeks of age). Coccidiosis rarely occurs in layers and breeders because of prior exposure to coccidia and resulting immunity in few instances to particular species. Outbreaks of any species may reduce or eliminate egg production for several weeks.

Transmission and vectors

Ingestion of viable sporulated oocysts is the only natural method for transmission of the disease. Oocysts can be spread mechanically by many different animals, insects, contaminated equipment, wild birds and dust. Oocysts are resistant to disinfectants and hence, it is difficult to stop spread by any disinfection measures.

Oocysts can survive in soil for many weeks but survival in poultry litter is limited to few days due to the ammonia production during wet litter conditions. The darkling beetles in litter are mechanical carriers of oocysts. Transmission from one farm to another is facilitated by movement of personnel and equipment between farms and even by migration of wild birds, which may mechanically spread the oocysts. Threat of coccidiosis is less during hot dry weather and greater in cooler wet weather.

Diagnosis

Coccidiosis can best be diagnosed from birds killed for immediate necropsy. Carcases after one hour after death are unsuitable for characteristic lesion as putrefaction in coccidiosis affected birds sets in quickly. Intestinal lesions of each part of the intestine (Duodenum, Midgut, and part of intestine and caeca) should be recorded with details to arrive at the correct 'species' diagnosis (see details of species specific lesions described previously).

Special diagnostic characteristics such as the large schizonts of *E. necatrix* or small round oocysts of *E. mitis* should be looked for to come at species diagnostic confirmation. Presence of few oocysts in faces indicates coccidiosis infection but not the 'clinical diagnosis of coccidiosis' which is confirmed only if gross lesions are serious and the economic parameters are threatened. Diagnosis should be based on findings of lesions and confirmatory microscopic stages on necropsy of typical birds from the flock.

Microscopic examination of small amount of mucosal scrapings diluted with saline on slide then covered with cover slip will be useful for diagnosis. Oocysts or macrogametes are most easily seen but the lesion is caused in many cases by maturing large schizonts, whose clusters in midgut are characteristic of *E. necatrix* while similar clusters of large schizonts in caeca is diagnostic of *E. tenella*. Method of 'Lesion scoring' is most useful in guaging the severity of infections.

Method of 'Dropping scoring' is also fairly useful in gauging severity of infections. For species identification based on 'Cross protection' test described previously in this chapter is used for research purposes. The oocyts can be preserved in 2-4% potassium Dichromate solution added to the faeces from infected birds and aeration of the faeces suspension, thus preserved can be undertaken for sporulation of oocysts at 37^{0}C overnight. These can be used for infection of experimental birds for identification test purpose mentioned above.

Prevention and Control of Coccidiosis

In earlier days, more emphasis on curative treatment of coccidiosis was given, using sulphonamides and other chemotherapeutic drugs like furazolidone and nitrofurazone for controlling coccidiosis outbreaks.

However, sooner the concept of preventive therapy emerged, as it was recognized that once the signs of the disease develop the economic damage is already set up in the flock inspite of the recovery of birds by chemotherapy.

In present days, almost all the broiler flocks receive preventive medication in the feed and treatment is the last resort if outbreak occurs. McDougal *et al.* (1986) has reviewed all the historical aspects of the chemotherapy.

Anticoccidial Drugs: Historical Aspect

In USA, Food and Drug Administration (FDA) approved various anticoccidial drug formulations time to time for undertaking preventive medication for control of coccidiosis as 'feed additives'. The following is the brief account of the same:

Sulpha quinoxaline (Sq, Sulquin) and Nitrofurazone (Nfz, Amifur) were approved by U.S. F.D.A. in 1948, followed by sodium arsanilate (progen) in 1949. Nicarbazine (Nicarb) was introduced in 1955 and Furazolidone in 1957. Terramycin (Oxytetracycline) was brought in 1959 while Amprolium (Amprol) and chlorotetracycline (Auromycin) in 1960 as well as Zoalene (Zoamix) in 1960. Combination of Amprolium + ethopabate (Amprol plus) was introduced in 1963. Clopidol (Coyden) was used for the first time in 1968 while Decoquinate (DecCox) and sulpha methoxine + ozmetoprin (Rofenaid) were used in 1970.

Monensin (Coban) was introduced in USA in 1971 by Elanco and was most popular for long time as preventive treatment for coccidiosis, Robenidine (Cycosta) was the product of American Cynamide Co used in 1972 initially.

Lasalocid (Avatec) was introduced by Roche in 1976 while salinomycin (Bio-cox) introduced in 1983 by Agri. Bio became most popular. Helofuginone (stenorol) was first used by Hoeschst Roussell Agril. Vet in 1987.

Narasin (Monteban) was a new molecule brought by Elanco in 1988 and Maduramicin (cygro) was brought by American cyanamide in 1989. Narasin + Nicarbazin (Maxiban) was introduced by Elanco in 1989 and semuduramycin (Aviax) was brought by Pfizer in 1995. New drugs pending approval in USA which are used in Europe, South America and Asia include diclazuril and toltazuril (synthetic Arianzines).

Mode of action of the anti coccidials

There are several (9 Nos) species of coccidia in poultry and all anticoccidial drugs have no effective action against each of these species equally. Each of the anticoccidial chemical compounds has its unique mode of action against coccidia. The sulphonamides compete for the incorporation of para Amino-benzoic Acid (PABA) and metabolism of folic acid. Amprolium competes for absorption of thiamine by the coccidia. The quinolone coccidiostats and clopidol inhibit energy metabolism in the cytochrome system of the coccidia. The polyether ionophores upset the osmotic balance of the protozoan cell by altering the permeability of the cell membranes for alkaline metal cations. This is how Maduramycin, Salinomycin and Monensin act.

These drugs act at various stages of the life cycle of the parasite e.g. The quinolones and ionophores arrest or kill the sporozoites or early tropozoites. Nicarbazin, robenidine and zoaline destroy the first or second stage schizonts and sulphonamides act on the developing schizonts and also on the sexual stages. Diclozuril acts in early schizogony with *E. tenella* but is delayed to later schizogony with E. *acervulina* and to the maturing macrogamete with *E. maxima.*

Some drugs kill the parasites and are coccidiocides while others only arrest the development and are coccidiostats. When medication is withdrawn, arrested parasites may continue to develop and contaminate the environment with oocystis. Relapse is possible in such cases. Hence, coccidiosidal drugs are more successful in practice.

Over dosing bring about toxicity of drugs of coccidiosis while underdosing brings about resistance. Long time use of anti coccidials will produce loss in sensitivity and eventually resistance. Drug resistance is a genetic phenomenon and once introduced in a line of coccidia, it will continue for many generation and hence continuous use of any particular coccidiostat should be avoided.

Continuous use of one single coccidiostat from day one until 3-7 days prior withdrawl of drug before slaughter is practiced for one broiler cycle. In broiler, maximum growth and feed efficiency with minimum disease is desirable while in layer or breeders, objective is immunization of birds.

The use of one product during starter feeding stage and another product in the grower stage is called 'Shuttle' programme. This improves the coccidiosis control. Continuous use of ionophore coccidiocidals may produce drug resistance and hence, it is now common practice to use Nicarbazin or halofunginone in either starter or grower phases to boost the anti coccidial control and take some pressure off of the ionophore. Drug resistance is reduced by 'Shuttle programme'. Rotation of the product is practiced by some, such as use of one product in 'spring' and another in 'fall'. Pullets which are started on floor during rearing are given coccidiosts only until they are removed to cages, when they mature and are then reared without anti coccidial drugs.

Immunization of birds against coccidiosis

Natural immunity after mild exposure is usually achieved by 2 different approaches. One approach is the 'controlled exposure' can be given by means of commercial products like 'Coccivac' 'Immucox' or 'Paracox'. This programme calls for a light harmless initial exposure followed by repeated two to three natural lifecycles. Careful supervision is required to provide adequate immunity. The second approach requires a natural exposure to important coccidiosis producing species (their oocysts) and a broad spectrum anticoccidial drug is fed to provide adequate immunity.

New Vaccines to prevent Coccidiosis

Precocious strains are developed now-a-days which can complete their life cycle fast with undergoing minimum numer of schzogonic cycles *in vivo,* when the pure oocysts of precocius strain of coccidia is fed to the bird under immunization. This brings about minimal or negligible damage of the epithelial tissue of intestine/caecum but the exposure of bird with this precocious strain makes the bird immune to the said strain. If multiple precocious strains are used for immunization (according to the most predominant natural strains of the particular poultry belt) immunity of multiple spectrum can be developed which can take care of coccidiosis as a whole for that area.

Precocious strains are produced by cultivation of coccidial cultures on choreo-allanotic membrane (CAM) of susceptible SPF egg embryos by serial passaging of specific eimerial oocysts and selection of those which have reduced their 'Cycle time' significantly which makes then to grow in smaller time very fast. This makes them do create minimum destruction of their substrate cells and, thus immunogenic with minimum creation of the cellular damage.

Coccidiosis of poultry, Indian Scenario

Where ever there is poultry, there is coccidiosis since ancient days. However, the coccidial unicellular parasites were not able to express themselves in the form of severe disease during the days of backyard poultry farming as heavy oocyst built up in littre which occurs on commercial poultry farms for precipitation of clinical disease was not possible in free range village poultry. The clinical coccidiosis became known to the Govt. and commercial poultry farms in early nineteen sixties in Bombay, Pune poultry belt and in the rest of Maharashtra.

Govt. farms introduced the regimen of drinking water medication (3-2-3 day treatment) using sulphadiamedine or Bifuran (Nitrofurazone + furazolidone) during nineteen sixties to keep the coccidiosis under control effectively which could avoid losses due to intestinal *E. necatrix / E. acervulina* infections) or caecal coccidiosis. Coccidiosis problem had increased tremendously in Bombay, Pune poultry belt during mid and late sixties due to immune-suppression caused by classical IBD in this zone after 1966.

Whenever there was rise in marek's disease problems corresponding rising incidences of coccidiosis were also recorded, such as during 1976 in north, during 1996-97 in Hyderabad and in Mysore during 1998-99, in Sangrur and Barwala district of Punjab, Haryana and Kashipur (UP) during 2005-06 in Panjab, Haryana and Hyderabad. It is difficult to say wheather immune-suppression caused by Marek's disease precipitates coccidiosis or coccidiosis precipitates Marke's Disease? Or both precipitate each other? It was noticed that coccidiosis when accompanies immune-suppresive problem, the most effective coccidiostat even fail to control precipitation of coccidiosis.

Cocciodiostats are added in commercial feed to control coccidiosis as prophylactic measure and when coccidiosis gets precipitated due to immune suppressive problems like CAA, Reo, ALC and Marek's Disease incidences, commercial feed gets blame. This happens even due to continuous underdosing of one particular coccidiostat in commercial feed. It is, therefore, necessary that the feed manufacturers should keep vigilance on field coccidiosis vis-à-vis coccidiostat and accordingly 'shuttle' the coccidiostats time to time for keeping coccidiosis under control but unfortunately this shutting is avoided by commercial feed manufacturers due to higher cost many times involved during this change. This point is observed by the author mainly in northern and eastern poultry belts in the country in recent years (2000 to 2007).

During late nineteen nineties, it was observed by the author in palladium and other broiler belts of south (Tamil Nadu) that there were paralytic leg reactions when farmers used monensin (coban) for anticoccidial preventive treatment in broiler flocks during first few weeks of the age of broilers. The investigation revealed that the farmers used Tiamutin (Tiamulin) also simultaneously along with monensin, for prevention of myco plasma (CRD) infection in the same flocks. It is known that 'Monensin' and 'Tiamutine' are contra indicated together as they invite paralytic neural reaction. The withdrawal of Tiamutin or replacement of the same with 'Tylan' for antiomycoplasma treatment improved the situation (problem was reduced and finally disappeared).

Coccidial live vaccines like 'coccivac' or 'Paracox' are tried in India by few progressive farmers but are not yet popular. Use of 'Precocious strains' for vaccination is still in infancy in India due to the high costs of imported vaccines.

However, the indigenous vaccine producer's research efforts are under progress and some vaccine may come out from the research projects of commercial vaccine manufacturers. But it must be noted that these vaccines, if made available in appropriate reasonable cost can be used and if adjuncted with chemoprophylaxis properly, may be able to effectively control coccidiosis in present immune suppressive scenario in poultry in India.

Suggested Reading

Johnson, W.T. (1930). Coccidiosis of the chicken with special reference to species. Stn. Bull. Ore. agric. Exp. Stn. 358: 3–33.

McDougal, L.R., Joyner L.P., and. Long P.L. (1986). Research in avian coccidiosis. Proc. Georgia Coccidiosis Conference, University of Georgia, Athens.

❑❑❑